Warrington and Halton Hospitals **NHS**

NHS Foundation Trust

Knowledge
& Library Service

"Bridging the Knowledge Gap"

This item is to be returned on or before the last date stamped below

@WHHFTKLS

whhftkls

http://whhportal.soutron.net

Tel: 01925 662128

Email: library@whh.nhs.uk

Medical Biochemistry at a Glance

For Lorraine and Saul

Medical Biochemistry at a Glance

BEN GREENSTEIN MRPharmS PhD
Director of Endocrine Research
Lupus Research Unit
Rayne Institute
St Thomas's Hospital
London SE1 7EH

Honorary Lecturer in Pharmacology
United Medical and Dental Schools
St Thomas's Campus, London

ADAM GREENSTEIN BSc (Hons)
Medical student
University of Manchester,
Manchester M13 9PL

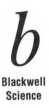

Blackwell
Science

© 1996 by
Blackwell Science Ltd
Editorial Offices:
Osney Mead, Oxford OX2 0EL
25 John Street, London WC1N 2BL
23 Ainslie Place, Edinburgh EH3 6AJ
238 Main Street, Cambridge
    Massachusetts 02142, USA
54 University Street, Carlton
    Victoria 3053, Australia

Other Editorial Offices:
Arnette Blackwell SA
    1, rue de Lille, 75007 Paris
    France

Blackwell Wissenschafts-Verlag GmbH
    Kurfürstendamm 57
    10707 Berlin, Germany

    Zehetnergasse 6
    A-1140 Wien
    Austria

First published 1996

Set by Setrite Typesetters, Hong Kong
Printed and bound in Great Britain
at the University Press, Cambridge

DISTRIBUTORS

Marston Book Services Ltd
PO Box 87
Oxford OX2 0DT
(*Orders*: Tel: 01865 791155
        Fax: 01865 791927
        Telex: 837515)

North America
Blackwell Science, Inc.
238 Main Street
Cambridge, MA 02142
(*Orders*: Tel: 800 215-1000
            617 876-7000
        Fax: 617 492-5263)

Australia
Blackwell Science Pty Ltd
54 University Street
Carlton, Victoria 3053
(*Orders*: Tel: 03 9347 0300
        Fax: 03 9349 3016)

A catalogue record for this title
is available from the British Library

ISBN 0-86542-980-4 (BSL)
ISBN 0-86542-626-0 (IE)

Library of Congress
Cataloging-in-Publication Data

Greenstein, Ben, 1941–
    Medical biochemistry at a glance/
    Ben Greenstein, Adam Greenstein.
            p.   cm.
    Includes bibliographical references
    and index.
    ISBN 0-86542-980-4
    1 Biochemistry—Outlines, syllabi, etc.
    2 Clinical biochemistry—Outlines, syllabi, etc.
    I Greenstein, Adam.   II Title.
    [DNLM: 1 Biochemistry.   QU 4 G815m 1996]
    QP514.2.G76   1996
    574. 19′2—dc20
    DNLM/DLC
    for Library of Congress   95-36168
                                                CIP

Contents

Introduction

Medical Biochemistry at a Glance was envisaged, designed and written as a learning aid for undergraduate students. The book consists of a series of progressively organized, self-contained two-page spreads, in keeping with the general formula of the 'At a Glance' series. The emphasis has been on the diagrams, with supplementary text, and an attempt has been made to keep the diagrams as simple as possible, given the immense complexity of the subject. We hope the reader will find the diagrams rapidly and comfortably accessible, and that they will give the information, literally, at a glance.

Although the book has been called *Medical Biochemistry at a Glance*, it has been written not only for medical students, and we hope that students of Biology, including nurses, will find the book useful. We have related biochemical function to disease, but the emphasis has been on the basic information and mechanisms. There are branches of Biochemistry which are not covered here. Plant Biochemistry, for example, is a very important and rapidly growing subject, as is Clinical Biochemistry, which deals in great detail with the biochemistry underlying disease, and with the measurement of clinical biochemical parameters in health and disease. It is hoped nevertheless that students wishing to specialize in those areas will find this book most useful as an introduction to Biochemistry.

Biochemistry is a vast subject whose knowledge base expands daily at an almost unbelievable pace, and this book, therefore, modestly hopes to cover only the basic information which underpins the progress that is made, and which will be required to ensure a good examination result for the student. The book is not to be thought of as an alternative to the substantial volumes of Biochemistry which are available, and which deal with the subject in far more detail.

We have made every attempt to guarantee the clarity, accuracy and reliability of the information, and have had the contents read by a number of medical students, whose comments and suggestions greatly improved the clarity of the diagrams. In addition, the book has been read by several experts, who have contributed immeasurably to the confidence with which we have produced the book. In particular, we wish to thank Drs Kathleen Rowsell, Richard Gregory, Graham Wallace and Ms Carolyn Watson, who read the entire book and made invaluable comments and suggestions. We are grateful, also, to Ben Bromilow and to Drs Gavin Brooks, Brian Ellis and Hywel Thomas for reading several of the chapters. It goes without saying, however, that any remaining errors (none we hope) are the responsibility of the authors, and if the reader spots any we should like to know.

It remains only to thank the editorial staff of Blackwell Science, and particularly Stuart Taylor and Jonathan Rowley, for their patience and guidance in bringing this project to a fruitful conclusion.

Ben Greenstein
London, 1995
Adam Greenstein
Manchester, 1995

1 The eukaryotic cell

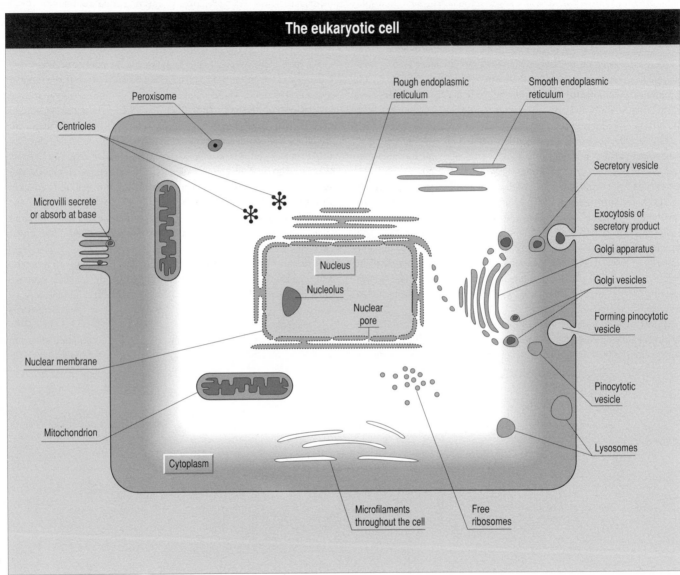

The eukaryotic cell

Peroxisome

Centrioles

Rough endoplasmic reticulum

Smooth endoplasmic reticulum

Secretory vesicle

Exocytosis of secretory product

Golgi apparatus

Microvilli secrete or absorb at base

Golgi vesicles

Nucleus

Nucleolus

Nuclear pore

Forming pinocytotic vesicle

Nuclear membrane

Pinocytotic vesicle

Mitochondrion

Lysosomes

Cytoplasm

Microfilaments throughout the cell

Free ribosomes

Fig. 1.1

INTRODUCTION

Eukaryotes have a membrane-bound **cell nucleus** with **chromosomes**, which are organized aggregations of genes. Algae, protozoa, fungi, slime moulds, plants and animals are eukaryotes. Prokaryotes are unicellular organisms, including bacteria, whose cells lack a nucleus and several other eukaryotic organelles.

Cell size

In animals, cells range in diameter from about 10 to 30 μm. Cells are usually microscopic to allow **diffusion**, a process whereby solutes distribute themselves in the available volume, and the rate of diffusion limits cell size. In most cells, no metabolically active region is more than 10–25 μm away from the cell surface. It would take days for amino acids, peptides and sugars to diffuse a couple of centimetres, but seconds to travel a few micrometres. Multicellular organisms have overcome this problem by developing a circulation.

INTERNAL ARCHITECTURE OF CELLS

The **cell nucleus** is bounded by two membranes: the inner, which defines it, and the outer, which is usually continuous with the cytoplasmic endoplasmic reticulum (ER). The nuclear membrane system is also called the **perinuclear envelope**. The space between inner and outer membranes is continuous with the lumen of the ER.

At points on the nuclear surface, the inner and outer membranes appear to fuse, creating **nuclear pores**, which may conduct materials between nucleus and cytoplasm. Most of the cell's deoxyribonucleic acid (DNA) occurs in the nucleus, as a DNA–protein complex called **chromatin**, which is organized into discrete, elongated bodies about 25 nm thick, called chromosomes. The DNA contains the cell's genetic information.

Inside the nucleus is the **nucleolus**, rich in ribonucleic acid (RNA). Within the nucleolus are one or more chromosomes, termed the **nucleolar organizer**, where ribosomal RNA (rRNA) is formed.

The non-nucleolar area of the nucleus is the nucleoplasm, within which occurs a small family of fibrous proteins termed **lamins**, which appear to bind DNA to the nuclear membrane.

Internal membrane systems of the cytoplasm

The ER is often the largest internal membrane system of the eukaryotic cell. Rough ER is studded with ribosomes, while smooth ER is not.

Smooth ER is the site of synthesis and metabolism of phospholipids and fatty acids. Smooth ER contains several enzymes that detoxify carcinogens or pesticides by rendering them water soluble and therefore more easily excreted. This may explain why some cells, such as liver hepatocytes, have more smooth ER than other cell types.

Rough ER is present in high abundance in cells that produce peptide hormones, e.g. insulin, and proteins, e.g. antibodies. Ribosomes bound to rough ER produce proteins, forming part of cell and organelle membranes. The rRNA–messenger RNA (mRNA) complex is attached to the ER, and usually passes the elongating peptide through a pore into the central lumen of the ER, where the chain aggregates prior to transportation elsewhere in the cell, or into the extracellular space.

The **Golgi apparatus** is a system of flattened vesicles and smooth membranes which transfers lipid precursors and carbohydrate to proteins to form lipoproteins and glycoproteins, respectively. The latter process, called glycosylation, is necessary for protein transport across the plasma membrane. The Golgi also produces much new cellular membrane in the form of vesicles, in which hormones, prohormones and some enzymes are packaged and exported from the cell. They also produce membrane for organelles such as peroxisomes and lysosomes.

Lysosomes are organelles with a single membrane, enclosing acid hydrolase enzymes in an acidic (pH 5) environment. The hydrolases degrade polymers such as DNA, RNA and protein into their monomeric units. The lysosomal membrane is impermeable to both large and small molecules, which are transported through it by specific mediators. Genetic lack of a lysosomal enzyme, β-N-hexosaminidase, which is important in the turnover of a membrane protein, G_{M2}, results in **Tay–Sachs disease** in which that protein accumulates in developing nerve cells and results in death by age about 5 years.

Peroxisomes are small organelles containing enzymes that use oxygen (O_2) to oxidize uric acid, D-amino acids and some 2-hydroxyacids, with the production of hydrogen peroxide (H_2O_2). H_2O_2 is converted in the peroxisome to water (H_2O) and O_2 by catalase. The peroxisome thus protects the cell from H_2O_2, a powerful oxidant. Peroxisomes also contain enzymes important in lipid metabolism. Peroxisomal enzymes vary from cell to cell, and with changes in cellular conditions. Absence of peroxisomes in brain, kidney, liver and skeletal muscle results in a rare autosomal recessive disease, **Zellweger syndrome**, which causes death within 6 months of birth.

Mitochondria are the energy powerhouses of the cell. They are large, being about 7 μm long and about 0.5–1.0 μm diameter, and may occupy up to 25% of the cytoplasm. They possess both inner and outer membranes. The outer membrane allows the passage of large molecules, up to 10 kDa, while the inner membrane is less permeable. The inner membrane has many infoldings or **cristae**, which protrude into the inner space or **matrix**. Respiratory enzymes protrude from the inner membrane into the matrix, as well as those which catalyse the production of adenosine triphosphate (ATP) from adenosine diphosphate (ADP) and inorganic phosphate (Pi). The matrix is filled with the enzymes converting acetyl-coenzyme A (CoA) to carbon dioxide (CO_2). Many substances, such as ATP, ADP, citrate and phosphate, which need to move into and out of the mitochondria, cannot pass passively through the membrane and are transported by permease proteins which form channels for them.

In the matrix are several copies of a small DNA molecule that codes for several key mitochondrial membrane proteins. Most mitochondrial proteins, however, are produced by cytoplasmic ribosomes using mRNA originating in the cell nucleus.

The **cytoskeleton** is a network of filaments and microtubules, which maintains cellular morphology, transport, mitosis, meiosis and cell motility. The microtubules are composed of polymers of the protein tubulin. At least three mechanochemical proteins, kinesin, dynesin and myosin, which convert chemical into mechanical energy, occur in the cytoskeleton.

The **cytosol**, where many reactions occur, contains soluble constituents. (Note: the **ribosome** is dealt with more fully on pp. 32–33.)

2 Membranes I

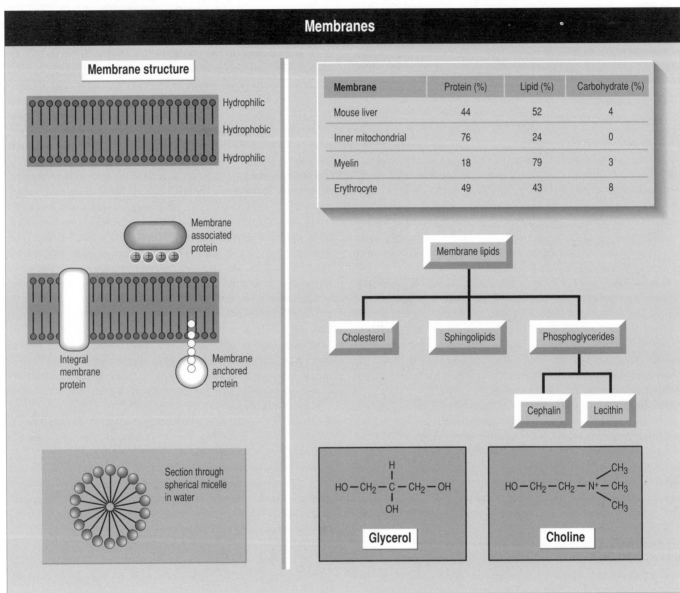

Membranes

Membrane structure

Hydrophilic
Hydrophobic
Hydrophilic

Membrane associated protein

Integral membrane protein

Membrane anchored protein

Section through spherical micelle in water

Membrane	Protein (%)	Lipid (%)	Carbohydrate (%)
Mouse liver	44	52	4
Inner mitochondrial	76	24	0
Myelin	18	79	3
Erythrocyte	49	43	8

Membrane lipids

Cholesterol — Sphingolipids — Phosphoglycerides

Cephalin — Lecithin

$HO-CH_2-\overset{\overset{\displaystyle H}{|}}{C}-CH_2-OH$
$\underset{\displaystyle OH}{|}$

Glycerol

$HO-CH_2-CH_2-\overset{\overset{\displaystyle CH_3}{|}}{\underset{\underset{\displaystyle CH_3}{|}}{N^+}}-CH_3$

Choline

Fig. 2.1

LIPID MEMBRANES

Functions

Membranes: (i) define the shape of an organelle or cell; (ii) control the exchange of solutes, e.g. sodium (Na^+), potassium (K^+) and chloride (Cl^-) ions between interior and exterior; (iii) form the site of chemical reactions, e.g. oxidative phosphorylation on mitochondrial membranes; (iv) are a site for recognition of chemical messengers such as hormones and neurotransmitters, whose receptors may be situated on the membrane; (v) have a role in cell–cell recognition; and (vi) facilitate cellular locomotion.

Architecture

All biological membranes range from about 5 to 10 nm in thickness, and contain protein and lipid, the ratio of the two varying with the membrane source. Mammalian membranes are especially abundant in phospholipids and cholesterol. The phospholipid bilayer is the common structural unit. Phospholipids are **amphipathic**, i.e. possessing both hydrophilic and hydrophobic portions in the same molecule. Hydrophobic interactions between the fatty acyl chains of the lipid molecules produce a phospholipid bilayer, a sheet or leaflet possessing two layers of phospholipids whose polar heads face the H_2O, while the fatty acyl chains form the hydrophobic interior. When phospholipids are shaken up with H_2O, they form spherical **micelles**, whose fatty acyl chains point away from the H_2O surface.

The lipid bilayer is coated on both sides with proteins, and according to the fluid mosaic model, the lipids themselves and some proteins move around in the plane of the bilayer.

The membrane proteins serve several functions. They may: (i) transport molecules through the membrane; (ii) act as receptors for chemical messengers such as hormones; (iii) make possible cell–cell interactions through their branching carbohydrate chains, which also make possible the recognition of antigens; and (iv) act as enzymes.

Proteins may be **integral**, being firmly bound to the membrane, or **associated**, being loosely or reversibly held to the membrane and able to be released by mild treatments. Integral proteins may be anchored, i.e. bonded covalently to the membrane by a link between the carboxy terminus of the protein and a membrane glycophospholipid (see below). Many integral proteins are insoluble in H_2O, and are embedded in the membrane and held to it by three main forces: (i) ionic interactions with the polar heads; (ii) hydrophobic interactions with the lipid interior; and (iii) specific interactions with cholesterol or other membrane molecules. Most integral proteins span the lipid bilayer and have polar regions at both ends of the protein.

MEMBRANE CHEMISTRY

Membranes are made up of protein, lipids and varying amounts of glycolipid and glycoprotein ('glyco-' implies a sugar moiety).

The three main lipids in eukaryotic membranes are **cholesterol**, **sphingolipids** and **phosphoglycerides**. Phosphoglycerides are the major membrane lipid components, and the two most abundant phosphoglycerides are **lecithin** (also called phosphatidylcholine) and **cephalin** (also called phosphatidylethanolamine). Sphingolipids are amphipathic molecules consisting of long-chain fatty acids with an amide linkage, which provides the polar head. Such a compound is termed a **ceramide**. **Glycosphingolipids** have a sugar moiety, either glucose or galactose, attached to the ceramide. Cerebrosides are examples of glycosphingolipids. **Galactocerebrosides** are cerebrosides found mainly in the central nervous system.

Cholesterol is a rigid molecule that intercalates among the phospholipids in the membrane. Its four-membered hydrophobic steroid ring interacts with the fatty acyl chains of membrane phospholipids. At 37°C, in eukaryotic cells, cholesterol limits the fluidity of the membrane. But, it also prevents the membrane from becoming less fluid at lower temperatures by preventing the chains from binding to each other. Membrane fluidity depends not only on the cholesterol content, but also on temperature and the lipid composition. Fluidity is promoted by shorter, unsaturated fatty acids. There is evidence that fluidity in membranes of certain cells may be influenced by diet.

THE ERYTHROCYTE MEMBRANE

The erythrocyte plasma membrane is relatively easily separated from other constituents. The lipid components are asymmetrically distributed across the membrane, in contrast to their symmetrical distribution in micelles. For example, cephalin occurs predominantly on the inner lipid layer. This asymmetry may be maintained by the transverse movement of phospholipids across the membrane, assisted by membrane proteins using metabolic energy to do so. An uncatalysed 'flip-flop' movement of sphingolipids and phosphoglycerides across the membrane is slow due to the tendency for the polar heads not to enter the hydrophobic bilayer, and may take days or weeks.

The erythrocyte membrane contains an integral glycoprotein, glycophorin, which contains 131 amino acids and spans the membrane, and another called **band 3**, because of its mobility on a polyacrylamide gel after electrophoresis. Band 3, a 900-amino acid protein, may have a role in the facilitated diffusion of hydrogen carbonate (HCO_3^-) and Cl^- across the membrane. It binds the cytosolic peripheral protein **ankyrin**, which in turn binds the protein **spectrin**. Spectrin and ankyrin are members of the erythrocyte cytoskeleton.

3 Membranes II

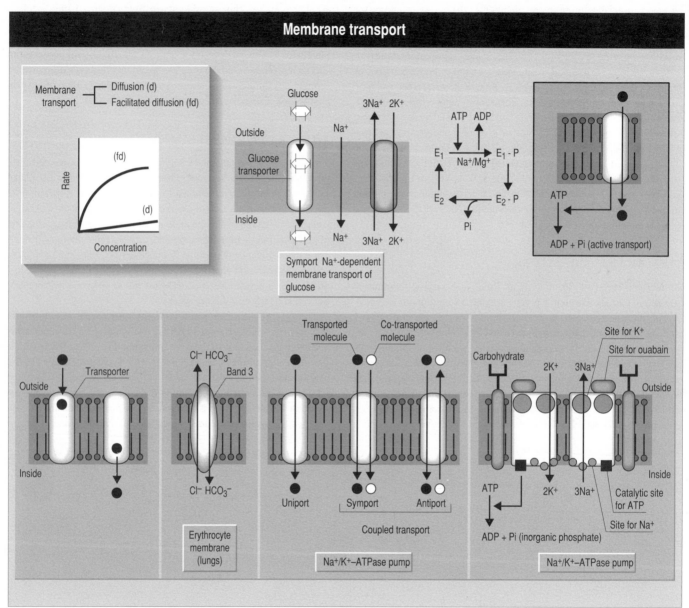

Fig. 3.1

MEMBRANE TRANSPORT

The membrane is selectively permeable to solutes in order to: (i) retain a barrier to the extracellular environment; (ii) ensure that essential molecules such as lipids, glucose and amino acids enter the cell, that these stay in the cell and that waste products leave the cell; and (iii) maintain ionic gradients across the membrane. Intracellular organelles may also have selectively permeable membranes. For example, the lysosome membrane maintains a concentration of hydrogen ions (H^+) 1000 to 10 000 times greater than in the cytosol. Transport across the membrane may be **passive**, **facilitated** or **active**.

Passive transport is the movement of a molecule or ion down a concentration or electrochemical gradient. It may be by simple diffusion, which is how gases such as O_2 and CO_2 and how a simple molecule like ethanol cross the plasma membrane. In simple diffusion, a small molecule dissolved in the extracellular fluid dissolves in the membrane and then in the intracellular fluid. The process is non-specific, and the rate-limiting factor for entry of the molecule into the membrane is its hydrophobicity, i.e. its solubility in oil. The rate of diffusion through the phospholipid bilayer is proportional to the hydrophobicity. It is also proportional to the concentration gradient across the membrane.

Facilitated diffusion is the rapid movement of molecules across the membrane, with the help of specific membrane proteins called **permeases**. The process is specific, is faster than would be expected from diffusion alone and there is a maximum rate of transport.

Active transport is the movement of ions or molecules across the membrane against a concentration gradient, which utilizes energy in the form of ATP hydrolysis to do so. There are three main types of active ion transport: (i) the Na^+/K^+–adenosine triphosphatase (ATPase) pump, which transports Na^+ out and K^+ in; (ii) the calcium ion (Ca^{2+}) pump (also called the Ca^{2+}–ATPase pump), which drives Ca^{2+} out of the cell or from the cytosol into the sarcoplasmic reticulum; and (iii) the proton (H^+) pump. Ion gradients generated by active transport can be coupled to the active transport of molecules such as certain amino acids and sugars ('secondary' active transport).

Cotransport is the transport of an ion or molecule coupled to a cotransported ion. **Symport** is the simultaneous movement of both in the same direction, while **antiport** is simultaneous movement in opposite directions. If transport is not coupled to a cotransported ion, the process is termed **uniport**. Cotransport may occur during facilitated diffusion or during active transport. Glucose can be transported by a symport-facilitated diffusion, while Cl^- and HCO_3^- are transported across the erythrocyte membrane by an antiport-facilitated diffusion pump called band 3, which pumps Cl^- and HCO_3^- in opposite directions, the direction depending on the prevailing concentration gradient.

Active transport requires energy generated by ATP hydrolysis to ADP, coupled to the pumping of ions against their concentration gradient: $ATP \rightarrow ADP + Pi$. Like facilitated diffusion, the transport is specific, has saturation kinetics and can be inhibited. An example is the primary active transport **Na^+/K^+–ATPase pump**. This is an antiporter enzyme system which requires Na^+, K^+ and magnesium ions (Mg^{2+}), and is present in virtually all animal cells, with especially high concentrations in excitable tissues such as nerve and muscle, and in cells actively involved in Na^+ movement across the plasma membrane, for example the kidney cortex and salivary glands.

The ATPase enzyme is an oligomer, composed of two α-subunits of 110 kDa, and two glycoprotein β-subunits of 55 kDa each. During ATP hydrolysis, the α-subunit is phosphorylated and dephosphorylated on a specific aspartate residue to form a β-aspartamyl phosphate. Phosphorylation requires Na^+ and Mg^{2+}, but not K^+, while dephosphorylation requires K^+ but not Na^+ or Mg^{2+}. The protein complex has been described in two conformations related to energy level, and the ATPase is thus referred to as an **E_1–E_2-type transporter**. The ATPase pump is inhibited by the cardiotonic glycosides, including **digoxin** and **ouabain**. Ouabain, due to its high H_2O solubility, has been extensively used to characterize the pump.

GLUCOSE TRANSPORT

Glucose transport provides an example of both facilitated diffusion and active transport, the former utilizing a uniport mechanism and the latter a symport mechanism. Glucose can be transported into erythrocytes by facilitated diffusion. The Michaelis constant (K_m) for glucose uptake into erythrocytes is about 1.5 mmol/l (i.e. at this concentration of glucose, about 50% of the available permease molecules will be bound to glucose molecules). Since the concentration of glucose in human blood is around 4–6 mmol/l, glucose uptake into erythrocytes will occur at virtually maximum rates. The permease is specific, since the L-isomer of glucose is not significantly transported into the erythrocyte. D-galactose and D-mannose are transported, but higher concentrations are required to half saturate the transport system. Once inside the cell, glucose is phosphorylated and can no longer leave the cell. The permease for glucose is also termed a D-hexose permease. It is an integral membrane protein of molecular weight 45 kDa.

Glucose can also be transported by a Na^+-dependent symport system found in plasma membranes of tissues, including the kidney tubule and intestinal epithelium. One molecule of glucose is moved against its concentration gradient, and one ion of Na^+ is moved down its concentration gradient by facilitated diffusion. But, the system is ultimately driven by the Na^+/K^+–ATPase pump. The symport is therefore a secondary active transport system. Amino acids are similarly transported.

THE CA²⁺ PUMP

The Ca^{2+} pump is an E_1–E_2-type active transport pump. It is an integral membrane protein, phosphorylated on an aspartamyl residue during Ca^{2+} transport. Two Ca^{2+} ions are transported for each molecule of ATP hydrolysed. In eukaryotic cells, Ca^{2+} binds to a calcium-binding protein called **calmodulin**, and the complex binds to the Ca^{2+} pump. Other Ca^{2+}-binding proteins include troponin C and parvalbumin.

4 Membranes III

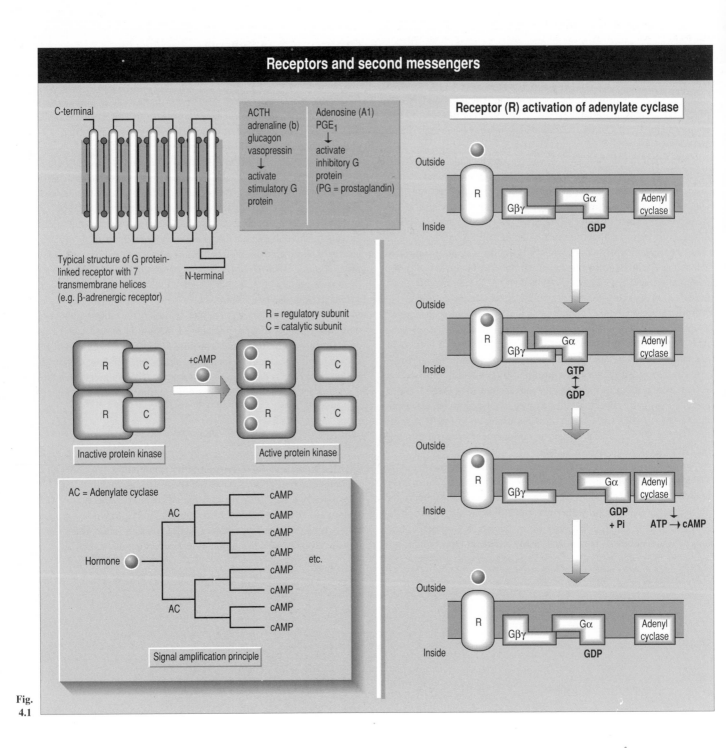

Receptors and second messengers

C-terminal

Typical structure of G protein-linked receptor with 7 transmembrane helices (e.g. β-adrenergic receptor)

N-terminal

ACTH
adrenaline (b)
glucagon
vasopressin
↓
activate
stimulatory G
protein

Adenosine (A1)
PGE₁
↓
activate
inhibitory G
protein
(PG = prostaglandin)

R = regulatory subunit
C = catalytic subunit

+cAMP

Inactive protein kinase

Active protein kinase

AC = Adenylate cyclase

AC

cAMP
cAMP
cAMP
cAMP

Hormone

cAMP
cAMP
cAMP
cAMP

etc.

AC

Signal amplification principle

Receptor (R) activation of adenylate cyclase

Outside

Inside

R   Gβγ   Gα   Adenyl cyclase

GDP

Outside

Inside

R   Gβγ   Gα   Adenyl cyclase

GTP
⇅
GDP

Outside

Inside

R   Gβγ   Gα   Adenyl cyclase

GDP
+ Pi

ATP → cAMP

Outside

Inside

R   Gβγ   Gα   Adenyl cyclase

GDP

Fig. 4.1

CHEMICAL COMMUNICATION

Endocrine signalling occurs when cells or organs release chemicals or **hormones** which travel in the bloodstream to target cells or organs, which recognize them through specific **receptors**. Receptors are proteins that may be situated on the plasma membrane or inside the cell. The receptor has sites that recognize and bind the hormone, and the binding reaction produces a change in the receptor which allows it to pass on to the cell the message that the hormone has bound to it. Examples of hormones are adrenaline, insulin, the sex hormones and thyroid hormone. **Paracrine** signalling occurs when the secreting and target cells are adjacent or close to each other. **Autocrine** signalling involves the release by a cell of a chemical that acts on the cell which released it. Growth factors are often paracrine or autocrine hormones. Sometimes, a chemical such as adrenaline, is both endocrine and paracrine.

Chemical signals or hormones acting on plasma membrane receptors are generally H_2O soluble (e.g. insulin, adrenaline) and produce relatively fast responses (seconds or minutes). Chemicals acting inside the cell are generally lipid soluble (e.g. cortisol, vitamin D), enabling them to pass easily through the plasma membrane. Their effects are slower in onset (hours or days) because their receptors alter gene expression and subsequent protein synthesis.

Receptors detect chemicals. They exhibit the properties of binding **selectivity**, high **affinity**, **reversibility** and **effector specificity** for the hormone that binds to them. An example of effector specificity is the action of adrenaline, which in liver cells causes glycogen breakdown and glucose release, while in neurones adrenaline may generate an electrical impulse.

Membrane receptors are integral proteins that span the membrane. On the extracellular surface is generally the N-terminal domain; inside the membrane is a helical hydrophobic ('H_2O-hating') domain; and the C-terminal domain extends into the cytosol. Membrane receptors may be linked to different signal transduction systems: (i) G proteins; (ii) ion channels; and (iii) enzymes.

A **G-protein-linked receptor**, adrenaline, binds to several different receptor subtypes, termed α_1, α_2, β_1 and β_2. For example, the β_2-adrenergic receptor recognizes both adrenaline and the neurotransmitter **noradrenaline**, as well as several artificial compounds, such as **isoprenaline**. The β_2-adrenergic receptor message transduction system has been relatively well characterized. The receptor itself has seven membrane-spanning helices, whose arrangement within the membrane may dictate the specificity with which the receptor binds the chemical. After the chemical has bound, the receptor interacts with other separate membrane components, which are the **G proteins** and the enzyme **adenylate cyclase**.

SECOND MESSENGER SYSTEM

Tightly bound to the cytoplasmic surface of the membrane is the integral **G protein**, so-called because it binds guanosine triphosphate (GTP) with high affinity. The G protein consists of three subunits, called α, β and γ, of molecular weight about 42, 35 and 10 kDa, respectively. The α-subunit can bind guanosine diphosphate (GDP) and GTP. The third protein integral to the membrane is the enzyme **adenylate cyclase**, which has an ATP-binding site on the cytoplasmic face of the membrane and, when the enzyme is activated, it converts ATP to cyclic adenosine monophosphate (cAMP).

In the absence of hormone, the G protein binds GDP, and adenylate cyclase is inactive. But, when the hormone binds to its site on the receptor, the receptor's conformation is changed and it binds the G protein. GDP dissociates, allowing GTP to bind instead. Consequently, the G protein dissociates into $G_{\beta,\gamma}$- and G_α-subunits. The G_α-subunit binds to adenylate cyclase, which is activated, and converts ATP to cAMP. cAMP is a so-called **second messenger**, relaying to the cell the fact that the hormone has bound to the receptor. Adenylate cyclase activation is rapidly terminated by hydrolysis of bound GTP to GDP, resulting in the resetting of the system for further stimulation.

Within the cell, cAMP initiates a cascade of protein phosphorylations by binding to a **protein kinase**. When cAMP binds to it, the kinase dissociates into two subunits, one regulatory and the other catalytic. The kinase is then able to phosphorylate other proteins by transferring the terminal phosphate group of ATP to serine, threonine or tyrosine residues of the substrate proteins. The end result of the cascade may be, for example, glycogen breakdown in liver or muscle, the hydrolysis of triacylglycerol to fatty acids and glycerol in adipose (fat) cells or the synthesis of steroid hormones in the adrenal cortex.

This type of cascade is an extremely efficient system for **amplifying** the signal, since the binding of a single adrenaline molecule results in the activation of adenylate cyclase molecules, and the generation of many molecules of cAMP.

Inhibitory G proteins also exist in the membrane, and these are activated to **inhibit** production of cAMP. They are activated by different receptors and hormones. These G proteins have $G_{\beta,\gamma}$-subunits, but a different G_α-subunit, called $G_{i\alpha}$, which binds GTP when activated, but which somehow inhibits adenylate cyclase. For example, adrenaline, through its β-receptor, stimulates cAMP production, while the neurotransmitter adenosine, through one of its receptors, the A_1-receptor, inhibits cAMP production. The adenosine A_2-receptor, however, stimulates cAMP production.

Note: cholera toxin, produced by the bacterium *Vibrio cholerae*, irreversibly activates G_α, so that it cannot hydrolyse GTP to GDP, resulting in continuously raised cAMP in the intestinal epithelium cell, causing a flood of Na^+ and H_2O into the intestinal lumen, massive diarrhoea and possible death from dehydration.

Other examples of second messengers are inositol trisphosphate (IP_3) and diacylglycerol (DAG), which are generated by activation of membrane receptors by hormones, for example through the action of adrenaline on α_1-receptors, or the neurotransmitter acetylcholine on muscarinic cholinergic receptors. The activated receptor binds to a membrane G protein, which stimulates the membrane-bound enzyme phospholipase C (PLC) to hydrolyse phosphatidylinositol-4,5-bisphosphate (PIP_2) to DAG and IP_3. IP_3 diffuses into the cytosol and binds to a receptor on the ER, which discharges free Ca^{2+} into the cytoplasm. The ions facilitate intracellular processes such as vesicle exocytosis or glycolysis.

5 Intracellular receptors and receptor antagonists

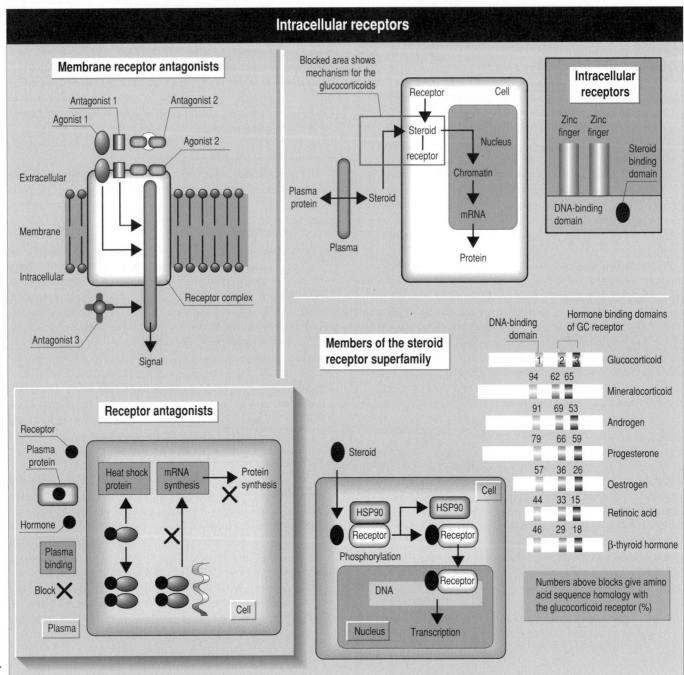

Intracellular receptors

Membrane receptor antagonists

Antagonist 1 Antagonist 2
Agonist 1
Agonist 2
Extracellular
Membrane
Intracellular
Receptor complex
Antagonist 3
Signal

Blocked area shows mechanism for the glucocorticoids

Receptor Cell
Steroid receptor Nucleus
Chromatin
Plasma protein Steroid mRNA
Plasma Protein

Intracellular receptors

Zinc finger Zinc finger
Steroid binding domain
DNA-binding domain

Receptor antagonists

Receptor
Plasma protein
Hormone
Plasma binding
Block ✗
Plasma

Heat shock protein mRNA synthesis Protein synthesis ✗
Block ✗
Cell

Members of the steroid receptor superfamily

Steroid
HSP90 HSP90
Receptor Receptor
Phosphorylation
Receptor
DNA Receptor
Nucleus Transcription
Cell

DNA-binding domain   Hormone binding domains of GC receptor

	1	2	3	Glucocorticoid
94	62	65	Mineralocorticoid
91	69	53	Androgen
79	66	59	Progesterone
57	36	26	Oestrogen
44	33	15	Retinoic acid
46	29	18	β-thyroid hormone

Numbers above blocks give amino acid sequence homology with the glucocorticoid receptor (%)

Fig. 5.1

INTRACELLULAR RECEPTORS

Intracellular receptor proteins bind to the lipophilic hormones which pass easily through the cell membrane. The intracellular receptors for **steroids**, **vitamin D** and **thyroid hormone** form part of a large so-called **receptor superfamily**, whose members bind to the nuclear chromatin and alter transcription.

Mechanism of receptor activation

The mechanism of intracellular receptor activation by hormone is not known, but there is evidence that in the inactive state, the receptor is bound by a **heat shock protein (HSP90)**. The number 90 refers to the size of the protein. The term 'heat shock' was given because these proteins were originally detected after cells were injured by heat shock, although it is now known that they are expressed in untraumatized tissues. There is a family of HSPs associated with diseases, fever, ischaemia, ageing and the inflammatory process. Some HSPs are also molecular chaperones (see p. 107).

When the hormone binds to the receptor, the HSP90 dissociates from the receptor, and the receptor proteins form homodimers. The receptor–hormone complex binds to specific sites on the DNA, called **hormone response elements (HREs)**, upstream from initiation sites. Many of the deoxynucleotide sequences of the HREs are known. Receptors for the sex hormones, and for glucocorticoids such as cortisol, are associated with HSPs, although receptors for thyroid hormone and vitamin D are not, and these receptors appear able to bind to their HREs in the absence of the hormone. In all cases, the process of receptor activation involves phosphorylation of the receptor, although the exact mechanism is unclear.

Nature of the receptor

The members of the intracellular superfamily of receptors contain three main regions. The first is a DNA-binding domain (region 1) which consists of two 'zinc fingers', so-called because each binds an ion of zinc (Zn^{2+}). This region is rich in cysteine and basic amino acids. It is believed that the first zinc finger determines the specificity of the binding of the receptor to DNA, while the other stabilizes the receptor to its response element on the DNA. Regions 2 and 3 of the receptor determine the hormone specificity of the binding reaction. From the scheme shown in Fig. 5.1, it can be seen that region 1 is very highly conserved among members of the superfamily, while the hormone-binding regions show much less homology.

RECEPTOR ANTAGONISM

The specificity of the binding reaction between ligand and receptor creates many opportunities for designing drugs that will lessen or prevent the action of the ligand. Receptor-blocking drugs play a large part in therapy, and examples include: (i) the β-receptor blocking drugs, for example, **propranolol**, used to treat cardiovascular disorders; and (ii) the anticancer drug **tamoxifen**, which inhibits the binding of the sex hormone oestradiol to its intracellular receptor, and is used in certain forms of breast cancer.

Antagonists can block hormone effects by binding directly to the receptor, or through indirect means. In classical pharmacological terminology, the ligand that activates the receptor is termed an **agonist**, and the ligand that blocks the action of the agonist is termed an **antagonist**.

Membrane receptor antagonism

In the scheme shown in Fig. 5.1, agonist 1 binds to its site in order to elicit the response, while antagonist 1 binds to an allosteric site on the receptor to block the action of agonist 1. An example of such an agonist–antagonist pair is the neurotransmitter **glutamate**, which binds to its site in order to open ion channels, and the antagonist **2-aminophosphonovalerate**, which binds to an allosteric site on the same receptor to which glutamate binds.

Two molecules of agonist 2 are required to bind in order to elicit a response, and antagonist 2 blocks by occupying the sites. An example of such an agonist is **acetylcholine**, which binds to two sites on the nicotinic receptor on skeletal muscle fibres. The antagonist **tubocurarine**, a muscle relaxant, occupies both sites, and blocks the action of acetylcholine.

Antagonist 3 does not directly antagonize the action of a ligand, but is able to penetrate the membrane and interact with the post-receptor mechanisms to block the action of the agonist. It may, for example, inhibit the passage of ions through a channel opened by the agonist. An example of antagonist 3 is the anticonvulsant drug **phenytoin**, which blocks the transmission of ions through the membrane.

Intracellular receptor antagonism

Intracellular hormone action can be antagonized by substances that interfere with the normal hormone–receptor interaction and post-receptor binding processes. The receptor itself may be blocked, or the post-receptor-mediated events, for example DNA binding, transcription or translation.

Dimerization block

Drugs have been developed that block the dimerization of the receptor once it has been activated by the hormone. An example of such a drug is the compound **ICI164384**, which appears to block the dimerization of the oestrogen receptor homodimers after they have been bound by oestradiol. (ICI is the company that developed the drug.) Failure to dimerize will compromise the ability of the receptor complex to bind to the HRE.

Transcriptional block

Transcriptional block is the mechanism whereby two important antagonists of steroid hormone action exert their effects. **Tamoxifen**, mentioned earlier, and the controversial substance **RU486** (developed by the company Roussel to block the actions of the hormone progesterone, and thus terminate pregnancy), both inhibit activation of transcription activation sites after they are bound by the receptor.

6 Molecules I

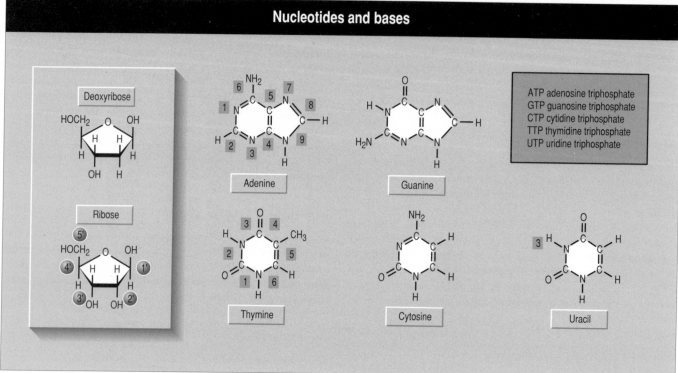

Nucleotides and bases

Deoxyribose

HOCH₂   O   OH

Ribose

HOCH₂   O   OH

Adenine

Guanine

Thymine

Cytosine

Uracil

ATP adenosine triphosphate
GTP guanosine triphosphate
CTP cytidine triphosphate
TTP thymidine triphosphate
UTP uridine triphosphate

Fig. 6.1

CHEMICAL BASIS OF CELLS

All cells depend on chemical activity, which can conveniently be classified in terms of **function and structure**. Functionally, cells rely on chemicals to provide energy, to maintain electrochemical gradients across membranes and to provide the messengers which convey information. Structurally, cells require chemicals to provide the building blocks for the structures which have been described in previous chapters, and for growth and repair of these structures.

Chemical size

Chemicals can be classified broadly in terms of size, as small or large molecules. Small molecules consist, generally, of less than 50 atoms, with molecular weights mainly less than 1000, and have been referred to as **metabolic intermediates**. They include the inorganic ions such as Na^+, sugars such as glucose, amino acids, for example glycine, nitrogenous bases including the purines and pyrimidines, fatty acids and steroids.

Larger molecules are called **macromolecules**. In the cell, the macromolecules are the **polysaccharides**, **proteins** and the **nucleic acids**. Macromolecules are composed of several smaller molecules, linked chemically by covalent bonds. When the smaller molecules are of one type, the macromolecule is called a **polymer**, and the smaller molecules are termed **monomers**. Thus, proteins are polymers, composed of monomers called amino acids. Monomers are also

commonly called **residues**. Nucleic acids are polymers of nucleotides, and polysaccharides are polymers of sugars. Some proteins contain polysaccharide moieties or groups covalently attached, when they are called **glycoproteins**.

NUCLEIC ACIDS

Nucleic acids are composed of nucleotides arranged in immense chains. Each nucleotide in turn is made of a base, either a purine or a pyrimidine, a pentose sugar (five-carbon sugar) and a phosphate group. The sugar is **ribose** or **deoxyribose**. When the sugar is ribose the nucleic acid is **RNA**. When the sugar is deoxyribose the nucleotide is **DNA**, and the nucleotides are deoxynucleotides. DNA, together with associated basic proteins called **histones**, makes up the **chromosome**. Humans have 46 chromosomes arranged in 23 pairs in the cell nucleus, and these contain the hereditary information of the body. The chromosomes have stretches of DNA, called **genes**, which code for specific proteins, as well as having associated sequences of deoxynucleotides which control the expression of the genes with which they are associated. A cell that contains two sets of the chromosomes is termed **diploid**, while a cell that contains only one set is termed **haploid**. Humans are therefore diploid organisms. The human germ cell, whether spermatozoon or unfertilized ovum, has only one set of 23 chromosomes, and is termed haploid. When the two combine during fertilization, the diploid status of the cell is restored.

Basic pairing of DNA

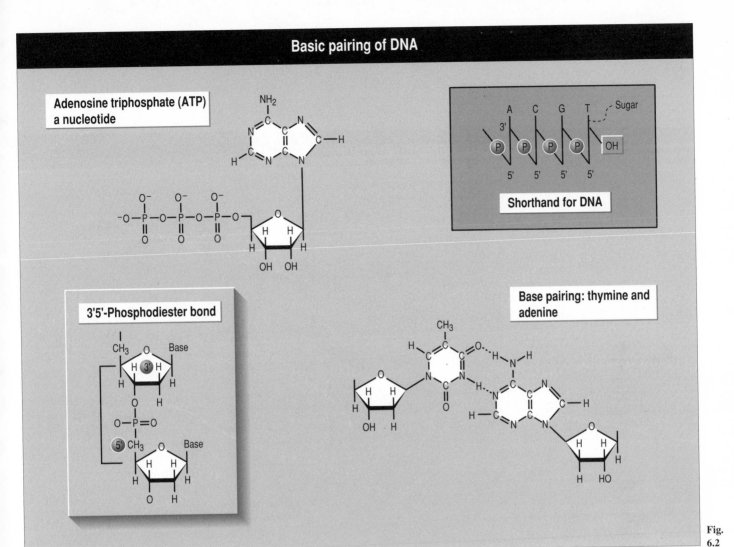

Adenosine triphosphate (ATP) a nucleotide

Shorthand for DNA

3'5'-Phosphodiester bond

Base pairing: thymine and adenine

Fig. 6.2

Nucleotide structure

For DNA, the bases of the nucleotides are ring structures, either **pyrimidines** (thymine (T) or cytosine (C)) or **purines** (guanine (G) or adenine (A)). For RNA, the thymine is replaced by uracil (U). For both DNA and RNA, the nucleotides are linked (or 'condensed') through the sugars, where phosphate groups link the 3' point of one sugar to the 5' point of another, releasing a molecule of H_2O. These phosphate linkages are termed 3'5'-**phosphodiester bonds**. In this way, a linear chain of nucleotides is built up. Because there are four different nucleotides, and because the chains can be assembled in any order of nucleotides, there are 4^n different possible nucleic acids having n nucleotides. For example, a nucleic acid containing 15 nucleotides has 4^{15} possible combinations (more than 1×10^6). The chain is represented as a strand with the 3' end having an unsubstituted hydroxyl (–OH) group on the left, and the phosphorylated 5' end on the right. During synthesis of DNA (or RNA), nucleotides are added to the 3' end.

Base pairing and the double helix

The DNA molecules in the cell consist of two complementary intertwined nucleotide strands. The strands are held together by what is called **base pairing**. When two strands of DNA come together, guanine will pair with cytosine, and adenine will pair with thymine through non-covalent hydrogen bonds. Thus, the base sequence of one strand will always be complementary to that of the other. Also, due to the way DNA is synthesized, the paired chains run in opposite directions; the 3' end of one chain lying adjacent to the 5' end of the other. Structurally, the chain forms what is termed a **double helix**. The double helix is a form of twisted or spiral right-handed staircase coiled round an imaginary central core, with about 10 bases every turn and the helix makes a complete turn every 3.4 nm. The double helix is held together not only by hydrogen bonding but also because the bases are planar and form stacks of base pairs held together by hydrophobic and van der Waal's forces (see Glossary, p. 112). The pairs can be made to separate simply by heating the DNA, when it 'melts' or denatures.

7 Molecules II

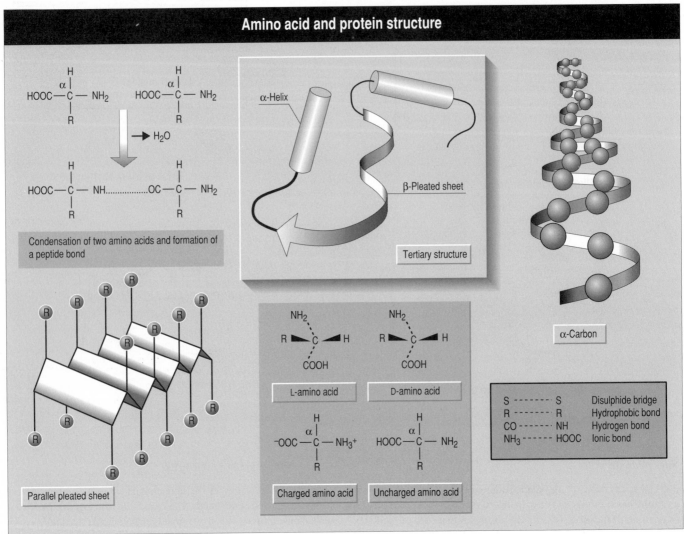

Amino acid and protein structure

Condensation of two amino acids and formation of a peptide bond

Parallel pleated sheet

α-Helix

β-Pleated sheet

Tertiary structure

α-Carbon

L-amino acid

D-amino acid

Charged amino acid

Uncharged amino acid

S ------- S   Disulphide bridge
R ------- R   Hydrophobic bond
CO ------ NH   Hydrogen bond
NH$_3$ ----- HOOC   Ionic bond

Fig. 7.1

PROTEINS

Proteins are polymers made up of monomers — amino acids. Proteins perform many functional roles inside and outside the cell, which also depends absolutely on proteins for its structure. Unlike DNA, proteins occur in many three-dimensional shapes, depending on their amino acid composition and arrangement. They may be fibrous (e.g. fibrin, collagen), globular (e.g. serum hormone-binding proteins), or antibodies.

Amino acids are so-called because all, with one exception, contain amino (–NH$_2$) groups. The exception is proline, which contains an imino (–NH–) group. They also contain acidic carboxyl (–COOH) groups. Chemically, amino acids have a common design: (i) a central α-carbon atom lying adjacent to the acidic carboxyl group is attached to (ii) the amino (or imino) group; (iii) a hydrogen atom; and (iv) to a variable side chain (R). At neutral pH, amino acids will be **ionized**, the charge depending on the relative numbers of amino and carboxyl groups. Lysine is positively charged, while aspartate is negatively charged. Some amino acids are more **hydrophobic** than others, depending on the hydrocarbon content of the R side chain. All amino acids, except glycine, have asymmetrical carbon atoms, and can therefore exist as **stereoisomers**. The two forms are mirror images, termed D and L, and proteins virtually always contain the L isomer.

Amino acids condense into polymers through the **peptide bond**, which joins the amino group of one amino acid to the carboxyl group of another, with the release of a molecule of H$_2$O. If the amino acid chain is less than 30 residues long, it is commonly termed a **peptide**, or **polypeptide**. Polypeptides can range in amino acid number from three (e.g. glutathione) to those which are made up of more than 1000 amino acids. Every polypeptide has a free amino group at one end, and a carboxyl group at the other. Proteins contain 20 different types of amino acids; therefore, a 200-amino acid polymer can have 20^{200} possible structures. This offers enormous variability in protein structure and function.

Proteins have four structural levels:

1 **primary** — the linear sequence of amino acids and the S–S bonds;

2 **secondary** — protein folding into α-helix and pleated sheets;

3 **tertiary** — regional folding between pleated sheets and α-helix, determined by non-covalent bonds; and

4 **quaternary** — non-covalent binding of different polypeptide subunit chains into a single protein molecule (e.g. haemoglobin, Hb).

Polysaccharides are polymers of sugars (also termed saccharides). Examples of polysaccharides are starch (storage form of glucose in plant cells), cellulose (part of plant cell wall) and glycogen (storage form of glucose in animal cells). Linkages can occur several different ways, and polysaccharides can occur in many different branched forms.

8 DNA replication

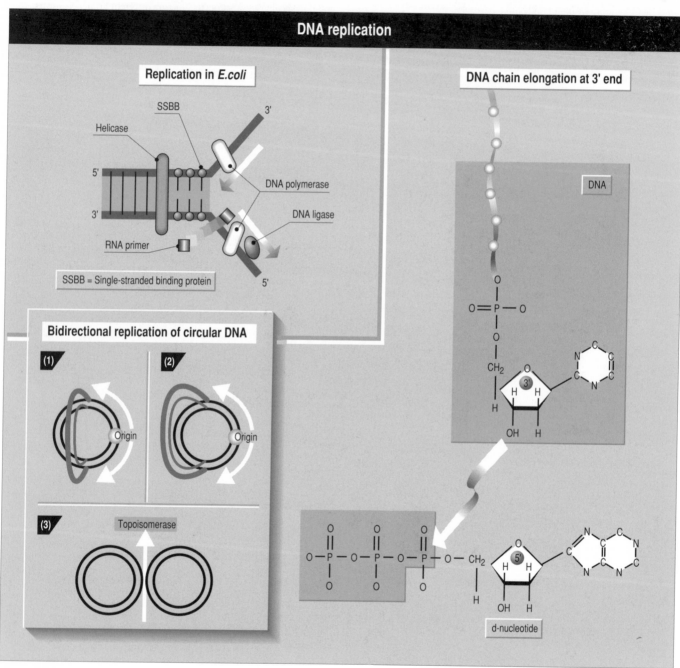

Fig. 8.1

DNA replication: (i) DNA chain synthesis; (ii) its initiation; (iii) termination; (iv) packaging with chromosomal proteins; (v) recombination; and (vi) DNA repair. A new strand of DNA combines with an old one. This is **semi-conservative** replication through **growing forks**. Replication is **bidirectional**, with both strands being copied. Each copied region is termed a replicon. Eventually, the replicons merge. In eukaryotes, the double helix is unwound simultaneously at several sites,

and replicated bidirectionally, until eventually all replicated stretches join up to form the new complementary DNA (cDNA) strand.

Unwinding is initiated by an appropriate cellular signal. A **helicase** enzyme system binds to a specific nucleotide sequence and unwinds the DNA adjacent to it to create a **replication fork**. The DNA is unwound just ahead of the DNA polymerase moving up behind to replicate the exposed strands.

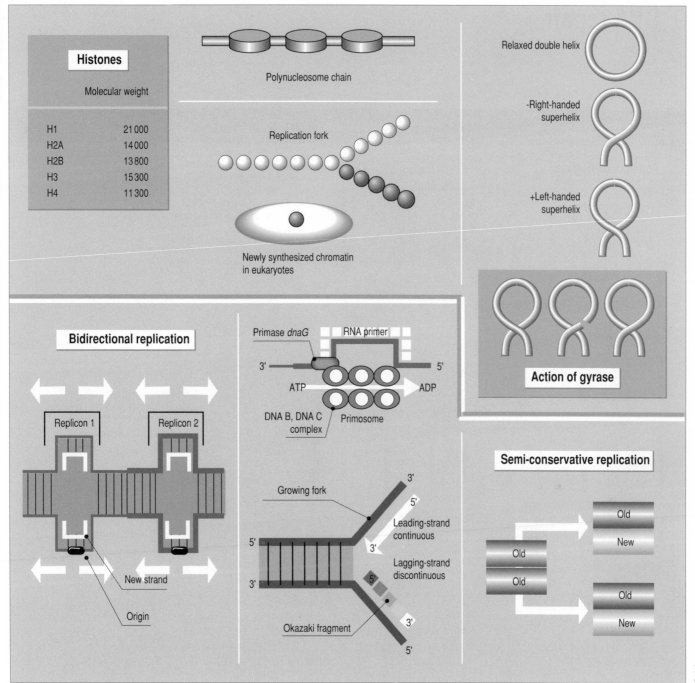

Histones

	Molecular weight
H1	21 000
H2A	14 000
H2B	13 800
H3	15 300
H4	11 300

Polynucleosome chain

Replication fork

Newly synthesized chromatin in eukaryotes

Relaxed double helix

-Right-handed superhelix

+Left-handed superhelix

Action of gyrase

Bidirectional replication

Replicon 1

Replicon 2

New strand

Origin

Primase *dnaG*

RNA primer

3'

5'

ATP

ADP

DNA B, DNA C complex

Primosome

Growing fork

3'

5'

5'

Leading-strand continuous

3'

Lagging-strand discontinuous

5'

3'

5'

3'

Okazaki fragment

Semi-conservative replication

Old

New

Old

Old

Old

Old

New

Fig. 8.2

REPLICATION

Replication is initiated by synthesis of a **primer** sequence of RNA at the starting point of replication on both unwound strands by **primase** enzyme activity of DNA polymerase α. (The primase gene is termed *dnaG*.) The polymerase begins elongation at the 3′ end of the primer. Elongation proceeds continuously along the 5′ → 3′ **leading strand**. On the so-called **lagging strand,** elongation must also run from 5′ → 3′, and runs in the opposite direction. Therefore, replication on the lagging strand is **discontinuous**, and has to stop periodically to wait for more of the strand to unwind. This creates segments of cDNA, called **Okazaki fragments**, about 100–200 deoxyribonucleotides long in eukaryotes. They are formed when proteins called **primosomes** attach themselves to the RNA–DNA complex and activate the reaction ready for the polymerase. After formation of the Okazaki fragment, the primers are removed and replaced by DNA, and the fragments are joined together by a **DNA ligase**. Errors in the matching of bases during elongation are detected by DNA polymerase δ, which 'proofreads' the bases.

Histones

In eukaryotes, DNA is associated with nucleoprotein histones. Their basic charge enables the histones to bind to the phosphate backbone of DNA. The **nucleosome** is a disc-shaped coil of DNA wound 1.5 times round a cluster of proteins including two molecules each of H4, H3, H2B and H2A. The **polynucleosome** consists of several nucleosomes joined by linker DNA. The **chromatin** formed from the DNA–protein complex is condensed into **chromosomes.**

9 DNA repair

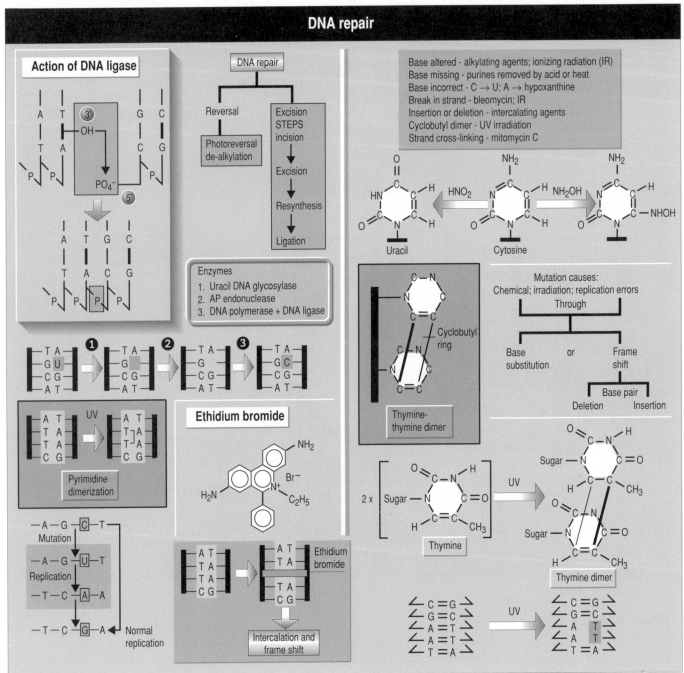

Fig. 9.1

DNA REPAIR

DNA repair is the maintenance of DNA stability through removal of errors in base sequence due to chemical or irradiation-induced damage, or through errors introduced during replication. Stability of DNA is essential for the preservation of genetic information. Survival of the species would be jeopardized by errors in rapidly dividing germ cells,

and cellular function would not be possible in stable cells, such as brain or liver cells, which may not divide for years.

In *Escherichia coli*, DNA polymerase I introduces on average one incorrect base per 10^4 base pairs. Genes in *E. coli* are about 10^3 bases long. Therefore, errors would be introduced every tenth gene (10^{-1} errors (or mutations) per gene each generation). But, the actual rate of errors is much less in *E. coli*: around 10^{-5} errors per gene each generation. It is thought that the rate of error production is similar in animal cells, which must also have a mechanism for repairing errors in coding regions of the genes.

Mutations can be defined as stable alterations in gene DNA structure. They may be **silent**, or **expressed** as phenotypic alterations. Mutations may be one of the following.

1 **Frame shift** mutations, which result from:
   (a) deletion of a base pair or block of base pairs;
   (b) insertion of new base pairs.
2 **Base substitutions**, which result from:
   (a) **transversions**, which are the substitution of pyrimidine–purine base pairs by purine–pyrimidine base pairs;
   (b) **transitions**, which are the substitution of purine–pyrimidine base pairs by pyrimidine–purine base pairs.

Tests for potential carcinogens include tests for their mutagenic effects on bacteria. This implies that alterations to DNA lie at the root of both carcinogenesis and mutagenesis. One test is the **Ames test**, in which a strain of *Salmonella*, unable to synthesize histidine, is grown in a Petri dish in a medium that lacks histidine. Any bacteria that grow are natural mutants. The suspected mutagen is added, and many mutants may be formed — some of which can synthesize histidine — and they will appear as yet more visible colonies on the agar. Different strains have been identified, some of which respond to mutagens that cause base substitutions, while other strains respond to mutagens producing additions or deletions, i.e. frame shifts. This makes it possible to identify, tentatively, the mechanism of action of the mutagen/carcinogen.

Repair is effected by **proofreading**. The proofreading ability of DNA polymerases was first discovered in *E. coli*. The enzyme DNA polymerase 1 is believed to have $3' \rightarrow 5'$ exonuclease activity, which enables it to proofread newly added base sequences, excise non-matching bases and replace these with the correctly matching bases.

Repair of pyrimidine dimers

Pyrimidine dimers are formed after exposure of DNA to ultraviolet (UV) light, when adjacent pyrimidine residues on a DNA strand may become linked covalently. The distortion of DNA produced by the dimer is detected by a group of proteins expressed by the *uvrABC* genes; the proteins consist of a tetramer of two proteins, P_{uvrA}, and two proteins, P_{uvrB}. The exonuclease enzyme P_{uvrC} cuts the strands at two places: four nucleotides away from the dimer on the 3′ side, and eight nucleotides away on the 5′ side. The excised 12-residue piece of DNA is unwound by a helicase P_{uvrD}, and diffuses away. DNA polymerase 1 moves into

the gap created, and uses the 3′ cut end as the primer and the intact complementary strand as the template to repair the cut strand. Finally, DNA ligase joins the 3′ end of the newly synthesized DNA and the original DNA.

Excision repair is also used by the cell to remove crosslinks formed by drugs used to treat cancer, such as cisplatin, mitomycin C and the nitrogen mustards.

> *Note*: *E. coli* contains an enzyme, DNA photolyase, which binds to the DNA region distorted by the dimer, and becomes photoactivated and splits the dimer.

Repair of deaminated cytosine

Cytosine may be deaminated to uracil, and this occurs spontaneously during the life of DNA. Since uracil can pair with adenine (U–A), the chemical change is potentially mutagenic. The presence of uracil on the DNA is recognized by uracil DNA glycosidase, which breaks the bond between uracil and deoxyribose by hydrolysis. The gap formed by removal of the pyrimidine is called an AP site (i.e. apurinic, containing no cytosine or thymine. The gap is recognized by the enzyme AP endonuclease, which cuts the DNA backbone adjacent to the missing base. DNA polymerase I cuts away the piece of deoxyribose phosphate and inserts cytosine opposite the intact guanine residue on the complementary strand, and DNA ligase seals the cut DNA strand.

Diseases associated with defects of DNA repair

These include hereditary retinoblastoma, Fanconi's anaemia and Xeroderma pigmentosum.

Xeroderma pigmentosum is the best understood. This rare disease is genetically transmitted as an autosomal recessive trait. Patients are highly sensitive to UV and sunlight, developing skin lesions soon after birth. The dermis atrophies, the eyelids scar and the cornea ulcerates. Freckles and skin ulcerations appear, followed by skin cancers.

The disease is caused by a defect of the exonuclease enzyme which nicks the DNA at the site of pyrimidine dimers, which are known to be caused by UV radiation. Skin fibroblasts from patients with Xeroderma pigmentosum have been shown to contain the deficient enzyme. Mutations in one of at least nine different genes can cause the disease. Although the incidence of the disease is low, about 1% of the population are carriers of at least one of the mutated genes.

10 Recombination

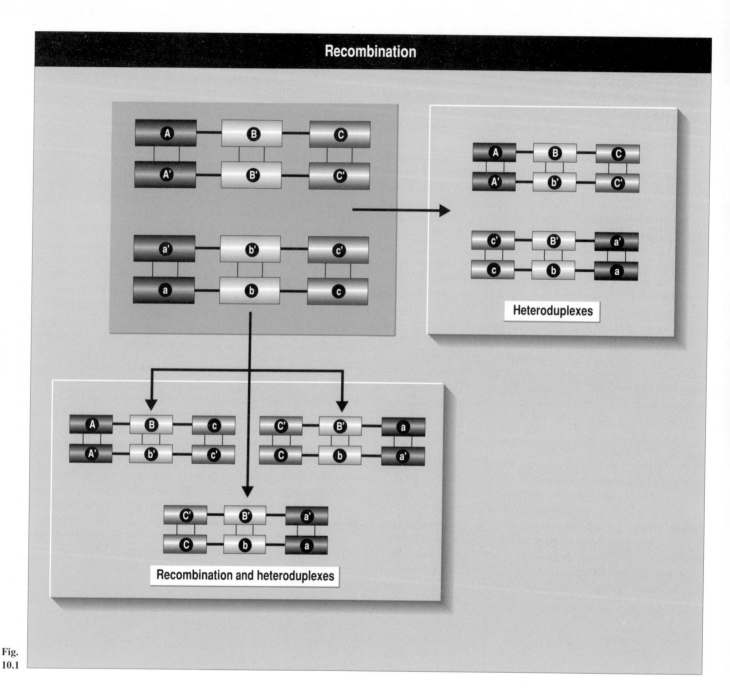

Fig. 10.1

INTRODUCTION

Recombination is the exchange or crossing over of blocks of genes by homologous chromosomes. Recombination takes place during meiosis in sexually reproducing organisms, and occurs in plants, animals and even in subcellular particles such as mitochondria and plasmids. The process involves: (i) the breaking of two homologous double-stranded DNA molecules; (ii) the exchange of both strands at the point of breakage; (iii) the exchange of genes; and (iv) the separation of the two altered strands of DNA. This process of formation of new DNA molecules is termed **general recombination**. When a gene is moved from one chromosome to another or from one part of the chromosome to another, this is called **transposition**, and does not require the same degree of homology as that for general recombination. The functions of rearranging genes are: (i) to repair damaged DNA; (ii) to generate new species of DNA, which is an important evolutionary event; and (iii) to regulate DNA expression.

MECHANISM OF RECOMBINATION

Initially, strands of DNA can join to each other by non-covalent base pairing to form **lap joints**, and these joints are made permanent by subsequent DNA synthesis.

ENZYMES OF RECOMBINATION

Single-stranded DNA for recombination is generated by a complex of proteins, P_{recB}, P_{recC} and P_{recD}, which are products of the *recB*, *recC* and *recD* genes, and which form a complex protein enzyme system. In *E. coli*, the complex: (i) recognizes a sequence — **5'-GCTGGTGG-3'** — the so-called *chi* sequence, and cuts the strand about four to six nucleotides away from the 3' end of the *chi* sequence; and (ii) the complex unwinds the DNA strands. The process requires ATP hydrolysis.

In *E. coli*, the **recA protein** utilizes ATP to catalyse the assimilation of a single strand of DNA into a duplex. The protein: (i) binds to the single strand, and the protein–DNA filament thus formed binds to the duplex; (ii) partially unwinds and 'reads' the duplex for sequences complementary to those on the single strand; (iii) further unwinds the duplex where complementarity and pairing occurs; and (iv) the exchange process continues along the duplex, and these are the mechanics underlying the process of branch migration mentioned above. All these steps require the hydrolysis of ATP.

SOS RESPONSE

Normally, low levels of P_{recA} are present in *E. coli*, due to suppression of P_{recA} mRNA production by a repressor protein termed P_{lexA}. P_{lexA} suppresses the production of many repair proteins. When DNA is damaged in *E. coli*, the cell initiates what is called an SOS response, generating hundreds of new copies of recA protein: (i) damaged single-stranded DNA binds to existing recA protein; and (ii) the complex formed binds to lexA protein and splits its alanine–glycine bonds, rendering it inactive. Note that P_{recA} therefore acts not only as a recombinase but also as a protease because of its action on P_{lexA}. Another gene activated by inactivation of *lexA* is the *uvrA* gene, whose product, the *uvrA* nuclease, cuts away thymine dimers which are formed by UV radiation damage.

MOBILE GENETIC ELEMENTS (MGEs)

MGEs, also called **transposable elements** or **transposons**, mediate the large-scale rearrangements that cannot be effected by general recombination. **Plasmids** are important MGEs confined to pro-karyotes. Plasmids are circular duplex DNA molecules which can replicate autonomously, and are therefore **replicons**. A replicon is any unit length of DNA which possesses its own origin of replication, and includes plasmids, bacterial chromosomes or regions of eukaryotic DNA.

Plasmids carry genes which express: (i) the generation of bacterial toxins; (ii) the metabolism of metabolites and other chemicals; and (iii) the inactivation of antibiotics. They are therefore tools of evolution and adaptation. Plasmids are also tools used by genetic engineers to introduce novel genes into cells. Engineers have termed particles such as plasmids, which are used to transfer genetic information between cells, **vectors**.

In recombination, plasmids may be F⁺ factor plasmids or R⁺ factor plasmids.

F⁺ factor plasmid

The DNA sequences of F⁺ factor plasmids ('F' stands for fertility) can be transferred between bacteria as follows.

1 A 'male' bacterium (F⁺) fastens itself to a 'female' bacterium (F⁻) by means of a **sex pilus** on its surface.

2 The pilus retracts to pull the two bacteria into close contact; one strand of the plasmid is cut and the DNA duplex unwinds.

3 The 5' end of the cut strand passes into the 'female cell', where a complementary strand is synthesized and a circular duplex plasmid formed.

The recipient cell is now F⁺, and the transferred plasmid has the genetic information required for production of a sex pilus.

The new plasmid can: (i) remain separate from the main bacterial chromosome; or (ii) become integrated into the chromosome, when the bacterium is now denoted as being a high frequency of recombination (hfr) cell. An hfr cell donates not just the F⁺ factor plasmid during transfer, but its complete chromosomal database. An hfr cell can splice out the F factor from its chromosome, and thus reverts to the F⁻ state.

F⁺ factor plasmids are not the only means of transferring genetic information between bacteria. This information can also be transferred by MGE called **bacteriophages**. A bacteriophage is a virus that infects bacteria.

R factor plasmids

These are so-called because they carry resistance to antibiotics. A bacterium can develop resistance to one or more antibiotics if it receives an R factor plasmid. The plasmid may contain a **resistance transfer factor** (**RTF**) as well as many so-called *r* genes. *r* Genes express enzymes that inactivate antibiotics such as tetracycline, streptomycin, chloramphenicol and sulphanilamide. Smaller plasmids, lacking an RTF region, will confer resistance to a single antibiotic when transferred.

11 RNA

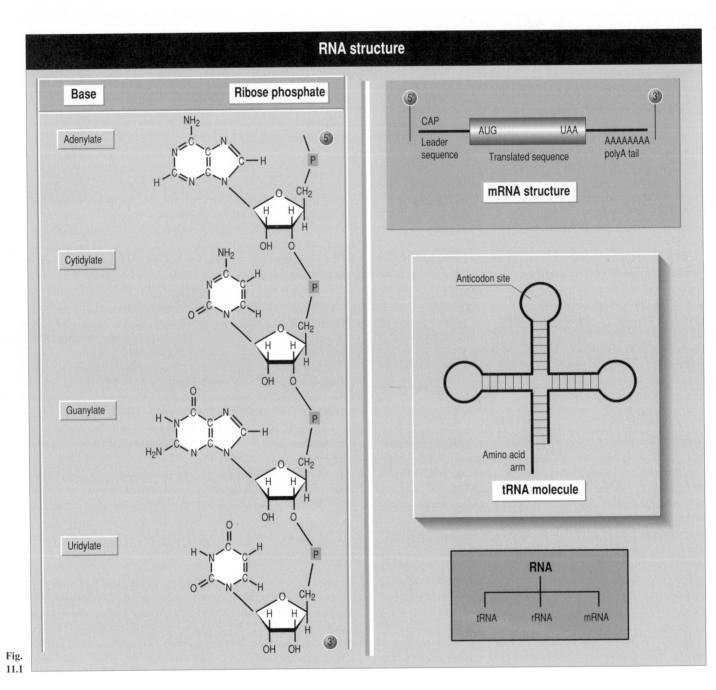

RNA structure

Base | **Ribose phosphate**

Adenylate

Cytidylate

Guanylate

Uridylate

mRNA structure

CAP — Leader sequence — AUG — Translated sequence — UAA — AAAAAAAA polyA tail

tRNA molecule

Anticodon site

Amino acid arm

RNA

tRNA   rRNA   mRNA

Fig. 11.1

RNA is an unbranched linear polymer whose chemical composition is similar to that of DNA, except that: (i) ribose is used instead of deoxyribose; (ii) adenine pairs with uracil (A–U) instead of with cytosine; and (iii) RNA exists as a single chain whereas DNA exists as a double helix. Two forms, transfer RNA (tRNA) and rRNA, may contain modified nucleosides, e.g. 2-methyladenosine, 5-methylcytosine, and there are several others. The base sequence of RNA reflects the base sequence of the DNA strand from which it was **transcribed**. In the case of mRNA, the information it carries enables the cell to synthesize, accurately, the proteins encoded by the genes.

RNA SPECIES

RNA may be classified in terms of its localization in the cell, its stability or its function. Thus, **mRNA** is the carrier of genetic information, **tRNA** is single stranded and carries the correct amino acid to the protein synthetic machinery and **rRNA** is part of ribosome structure.

mRNA

mRNA may be **monocistronic** or **polycistronic**. Eukaryotic mRNA is monocistronic, i.e. one mRNA molecule carries information about one protein only, whereas a prokaryotic mRNA molecule may be polycistronic, carrying information about more than one protein. mRNA is relatively unstable, being broken down rapidly after transcription has occurred. Some forms of mRNA may be stored in an inactive form until required, for example in amphibian ova or unfertilized eggs, where they remain 'silent' until fertilization. Structurally, mRNA differs from other forms of RNA because of its function as a template for **translation** into protein. At the 5′ end of the linear mRNA is a 'cap', made of a 7-methylated guanosine-5′-triphosphate. The cap prevents phosphatases and nucleases from metabolizing the 5′ end of the mRNA, and also serves as a recognition site for the ribosomal initiation factor (see p. 33). (Note, however, that 5-methylated cytidines and 6-methylated adenosines have been discovered further along the strand.) Following the cap is a **leader sequence**, and after this the **initiation codon** (see p. 32) or sequence, most commonly adenine–uracil–guanine (**AUG**). Following this is the coding region, whose message is ended by a **termination codon** which may be **UGA**, **UUA** or **UAG**. At the 3′ end is a non-translated **trailer sequence**, followed by a polyadenylated (polyA) tail, whose role is not known, but which may enhance stability.

rRNA

rRNA constitutes about 80% of total cellular RNA and is stable metabolically, mainly because of its association with the ribosomal proteins. The eukaryotic ribosome is made up of two subunits, the 40S subunit, and the 60S subunit. (Note: S is the Svedberg unit, which gives an indication of the relative size and molecular weight of a macromolecule.) The two subunits together contain around 75 proteins and four different species of rRNA, distinguished by size. The 40S subunit contains just over 50% of the protein and a molecule of 18S rRNA. The 60S subunit contains the rest of the protein, and a 5S, 5.8S and 28S rRNA. The 5S, 18S and 28S are synthesized in the nucleolus, and the 5S in the nucleoplasm.

rRNA molecules assume secondary structuring, forming base pairs within the molecule, allowing formation of helical regions. RNA may also form so-called hairpin loops. The conformations and nucleotide sequence of 5S, for example, are remarkably constant in evolutionary terms, being very similar in *E. coli* and humans. If the ribosome lacks 5S it cannot translate mRNA into protein. The large rRNA forms contain several modified nucleotides, particularly 2′-methylations on ribose, and several methylations of the bases, which may be necessary for processing RNA precursors.

> *Note*: methylation of bases in rRNA can confer resistance to antibiotics in bacteria. For example, *Staphylococcus aureus* can develop resistance to lincomycin and erythromycin if it acquires a plasmid that carries the gene coding for a methylase, which N6-methylates adenosine on 23S rRNA. This blocks the binding of erythromycin to the large bacterial ribosomal subunit.

rRNA may mediate translation by pairing with specific regions of mRNA, and by operating, together with the proteins, the hinging apparatus of the ribosome.

tRNA

tRNA constitutes around 15% of the total cellular RNA, and has several functions:

1 it binds specific amino acids, thereby raising their activity levels for formation of peptide bonds;

2 it carries the amino acid to the polyribosome; and

3 it accurately recognizes the correct codon in the mRNA, corresponding to the amino acid it carries.

One tRNA molecule carries one species only of amino acid, and although there are 20 amino acids, there are over 50 different species of tRNA in the cell. An amino acid may be able to bind to more than one species of tRNA, which are called **isoacceptors**.

tRNA has two active sites: (i) at the 3′ end –CCA–OH, to which the amino acid is enzymatically attached (if, for example, the tRNA carries arginine, it is called tRNA^{Arg}); and (ii) an **anticodon triplet**, which recognizes the complementary codon on the mRNA at the ribosomal complex.

Structurally, tRNA forms the so-called **clover leaf** secondary structure through base pairing; the anticodon active site is situated on one of the clover leaves, and the –CCA–OH site on the stem. There are several modified bases in tRNA, although their precise function is not known. They may be involved in tRNA–protein interactions and in enhancing tRNA stability.

RNA type	Site synthesized, S units*	Function
Messenger RNA (mRNA)	Nucleoplasm	Template for protein synthesis
Transfer RNA (tRNA)	Nucleoplasm 4S	Transfers amino acids to mRNA
Small nuclear RNA (snRNA)	Nucleoplasm	Chromatin regulatory and structural RNA
Heterogeneous nuclear RNA (hnRNA)	Nucleoplasm 30–100S	Precursors of other RNA
Ribosomal RNA (rRNA)	Nucleoplasm 5S	Part of ribosome structure
	Nucleolus 5.9–18S	
	Mitochondria 12–16S	
Mitochondrial mRNA (mt mRNA)	Mitochondria 9–40S	Template for protein synthesis
Mitochondrial tRNA (mt tRNA)	Mitochondria 3.2–4S	Transfers amino acids to mRNA
Small cytoplasmic RNA (scRNA)	Rough ER and cytosol 7S	Selects protein for export

* S, Svedberg units; coefficient of sedimentation.

12 Transcription I

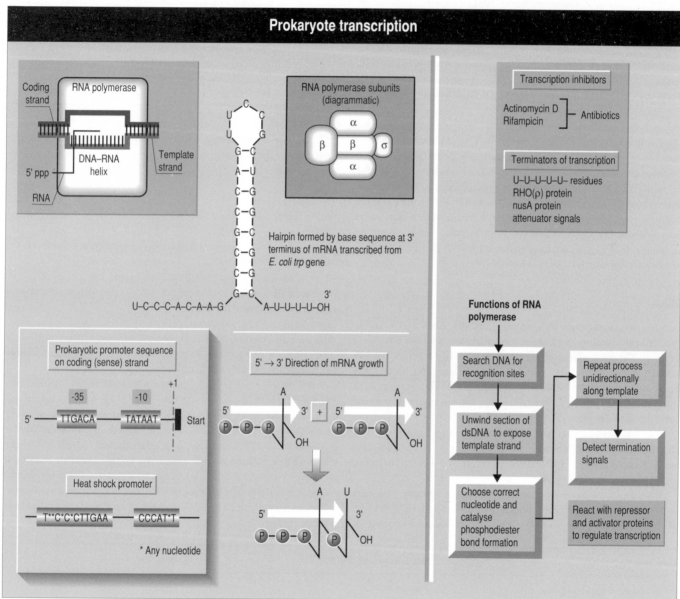

Prokaryote transcription

Coding strand — RNA polymerase — Template strand

DNA–RNA helix

5′ ppp

RNA

RNA polymerase subunits (diagrammatic)

α
β β σ
α

Hairpin formed by base sequence at 3′ terminus of mRNA transcribed from *E. coli trp* gene

U–C–C–C–A–C–A–A–G — A–U–U–U–U–OH 3′

Transcription inhibitors

Actinomycin D
Rifampicin — Antibiotics

Terminators of transcription

U–U–U–U–U– residues
RHO(ρ) protein
nusA protein
attenuator signals

Prokaryotic promoter sequence on coding (sense) strand

-35   -10   +1

5′ — TTGACA — TATAAT — Start

Heat shock promoter

— T**C*C*CTTGAA — CCCAT*T —

* Any nucleotide

5′ → 3′ Direction of mRNA growth

Functions of RNA polymerase

Search DNA for recognition sites

Unwind section of dsDNA to expose template strand

Choose correct nucleotide and catalyse phosphodiester bond formation

Repeat process unidirectionally along template

Detect termination signals

React with repressor and activator proteins to regulate transcription

Fig. 12.1

RNA molecules are synthesized in the cell by RNA polymerases, which catalyse the formation of linear polynucleotides whose sequence is complementary to the DNA template. RNA is synthesized from the 5′ to the 3′ end. In prokaryotes, for example *E. coli*, from which much of the information about transcription has been obtained, RNA is synthesized in the cytoplasm and immediately used as a template for protein synthesis.

PROKARYOTES

In *E. coli*, transcription occurs in three phases: (i) initiation; (ii) elongation; and (iii) termination, and is catalysed by a single RNA polymerase, consisting of four subunits: $\alpha_2\beta\beta'\sigma$, and the complete enzyme is termed a **holoenzyme**. The subunits have different functions: σ identifies the promoter site, initiates transcription, and thereafter dissociates from the enzyme; β′ binds to the DNA template; and β binds the nucleotides. The functions of the two α-subunits are not known. $\alpha_2\beta\beta'$ is called the core enzyme, and contains the catalytic site.

The σ-subunit quickly enables RNA polymerase to identify the promoter region, without the need for the double helix to be unwound; it also decreases the affinity of the enzyme for non-specific regions of the DNA molecule.

Promoter sites

Promoters are short sequences on the coding strand (as opposed to the template strand) upstream, i.e. on the 5′ side, of the **start site** of RNA synthesis. Two promoters have been identified in *E. coli*: the −35 and the −10 (Pribnow box) sequences, separated from each other, optimally, by 25 bases. If either of these sequences is altered by one base, the promoter loses most if not all activity.

Heat shock prompts *E. coli* to produce several HSPs, which help it to cope with the heat trauma. This occurs because the cell rapidly produces a different type of σ-unit called σ^{32}; σ^{32} recognizes a different set of promoters.

DNA unwinding and RNA synthesis

When RNA polymerase binds to the correct section of the double helix, it unwinds a 17-base-pair-long section of DNA, corresponding to 1.6 turns of the helix. Unlike DNA synthesis, RNA synthesis can begin without a primer. RNA synthesis proceeds from 5′ to 3′ end (similar to DNA synthesis), and at the 5′ end of the newly synthesized RNA is invariably found pppA or pppG (p, phosphate). At the free 3′ end (or terminus) is a free −OH group. The newly formed RNA is called **nascent RNA**; nascent means newborn, but not yet active. The complex consisting of the nascent RNA, the RNA polymerase and the portion of unwound DNA is sometimes called the **transcription bubble**. In *E. coli*, the speed of transcription is around 50 nucleotides incorporated into nascent RNA per second, and during this period the bubble moves 17 nm along the DNA. As the bubble moves along, unwinding the helix, so the helix is rewound at the same rate after the bubble has passed. Unlike DNA polymerase, RNA polymerase does not proofread or alter any errors (i.e. edit) of the newly synthesized RNA. Therefore, the error rate is greater than for DNA synthesis; DNA polymerase may make errors once every 10^{10} bases, whereas RNA polymerase may make errors once every 10^5 bases.

Termination of transcription

Transcription is terminated when RNA polymerase encounters **stop signals** on the DNA template strand. For example, on the DNA template of the *trp* gene of *E. coli* is a **palindromic** length rich in GC bases, followed by one rich in AT bases. The term 'palindrome' refers to a sequence of bases that is identical when read from left to right, or from right to left, e.g. TAAT or GCCG. The RNA bases corresponding to this stretch of DNA spontaneously assume the so-called **hairpin** structure. After the hairpin, a series of U bases (uridine triphosphate, UTP) are added. Shortly after this addition: (i) RNA polymerase stops; (ii) the nascent RNA dissociates from the bubble; and (iii) the DNA reforms the double helix.

> *Note*: RNA polymerase activity is inhibited by the hairpin structure, and the series of U bases forms an especially weak pairing with the template strand. This facilitates dissociation of RNA from the DNA template.

There is in *E. coli*, a protein called **nusA** protein that terminates transcription. There are also **attenuator sites** on some *E. coli* genes that terminate transcription.

The **ρ (Rho) factor** is an enzyme, found in some phage particles, that hydrolyses ATP in the presence of single-stranded RNA, and which binds newly formed RNA. ρ acts as a terminator of transcription by using the energy from hydrolysis of ATP to move along the nascent RNA towards the bubble, and it pulls RNA away from the bubble when it reaches a certain signal in the RNA molecule itself. As with ρ-independent termination of transcription, the termination signal resides in the RNA and not on the DNA template.

Post-transcription processing

In prokaryotes, there is very little if any post-transcriptional processing of mRNA. But, rRNA and tRNA nascent chains are cleaved and some of their bases are modified.

1 One nascent chain may be cleaved by enzymes called **nucleases** to yield several species of tRNA and rRNA.

2 Another modification is the addition of terminal nucleotides at the 3′ end. For example, tRNA receives the sequence CCA at the 3′ end (see p. 23).

3 Molecules of rRNA may be altered by methylation of bases.

Inhibition of transcription

Transcription can be inhibited using drugs, for example some antibiotics.

Rifampicin reacts with the β-subunit of RNA polymerase to block the first phosphodiester bond between nucleotides. But, if transcription has started, rifampicin is ineffective. Bacteria can develop resistance to rifampicin by producing a mutated β-subunit, when they are termed *rif-r* mutants.

A molecule of **actinomycin D** intercalates between two GC pairs of double-helical DNA in the narrow groove of the helix. Actinomycin D does not bind to the RNA–DNA duplex, nor does it bind to single-stranded DNA or RNA.

13 Transcription II

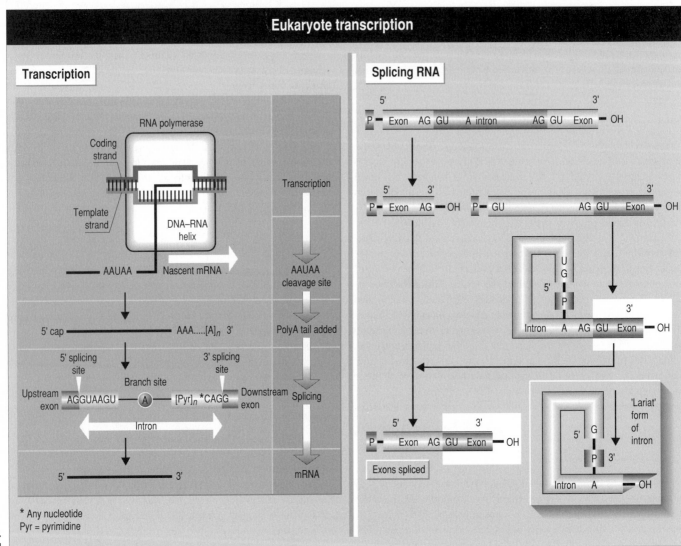

Transcription

RNA polymerase
Coding strand
Template strand
DNA–RNA helix
AAUAA   Nascent mRNA

5' cap —— AAA.....[A]$_n$ 3'

5' splicing site   Branch site   3' splicing site
Upstream exon   AGGUAAGU (A) [Pyr]$_n$ *CAGG   Downstream exon
Intron

5' ——————— 3'

Transcription
AAUAA cleavage site
PolyA tail added
Splicing
mRNA

* Any nucleotide
Pyr = pyrimidine

Splicing RNA

5' P — Exon AG GU A intron AG GU Exon — OH 3'

5' P — Exon AG — OH   P — GU   AG GU Exon — OH 3'

U G
5' P
Intron A AG GU Exon — OH 3'

5' P — Exon AG GU Exon — OH 3'
Exons spliced

'Lariat' form of intron
5' G P 3'
Intron A — OH

Fig. 13.1

EUKARYOTIC TRANSCRIPTION

Eukaryotic transcription occurs inside the nucleus, and the transcribed mRNA is translated outside the nucleus. In eukaryotes, there are three different types of RNA polymerase, and the nascent RNA formed is extensively processed before being utilized by the cell. In particular, the RNA is **spliced**, and the nature of the splicing depends on the function of the RNA. In eukaryotes, mRNA is derived from heterogeneous nuclear RNA (hnRNA; the primary transcript), which is extensively hydrolysed within the nucleus.

RNA polymerase

Transcription is initiated without the need for a primer, and mRNA is synthesized by addition of nucleoside triphosphates in the direction $5' \rightarrow 3'$.

Species	Nuclear localization	RNA products
I	Nucleolus	**rRNA**: 5.8S, 18S, 28S
II	Nucleoplasm*	**mRNA**: hnRNA and mRNA precursors
III	Nucleoplasm	**rRNA**: 5S; **tRNA**

* Strongly inhibited by low doses of the fungal toxin α-amanitin. (III is blocked by higher doses of α-amanitin; I is insensitive.)

EUKARYOTIC PROMOTERS

As in prokaryotes, RNA polymerase recognizes promoter sequences upstream of the start site, but polymerases I, II and III recognize different start sites. RNA polymerase II requires three start sites: at –110 is the

CAAT box (CA–CAATC); at –40 is the **GC box** (GGGCGG); at –25 is the **TATA box**, also called the **Hogness box** (TATAAA). The CAAT box aids the binding of polymerase II to the DNA, and the TATA box guides polymerase II to the correct start site. The GC box is most often found on constitutive genes (continuously expressed), rather than on those which are, for example, developmentally regulated.

In addition to promoters, there are **enchancer sequences** which may be thousands of bases away from the start site, either upstream, downstream or both, and may be on either coding or template strands of the DNA. Enhancers on their own, however, are not promoters. Enhancers may confer **specificity** of cellular or organ responses to chemical stimuli. They have sites that bind sets of protein modifiers, both positive or negative in action. Steroid and thyroid hormones, for example, bind to intracellular receptors which in turn bind to enhancers, thus initiating transcription. Only those cells that normally contain the receptors and/or the enhancers will respond to the chemical stimulus.

TRANSCRIPTION FACTORS

Transcription factors are proteins that are required in order for RNA polymerase to recognize promoter sites. For example, genes containing GC boxes require a protein termed **spl**. A transcription factor called **CTF** binds to the CAAT box, and a protein, **B protein**, discovered in *Drosophila*, binds to the TATA box.

The **5′ cap** is added to the 5′ end of eukaryotic mRNA very soon after transcription is initiated. The cap has at least three functions:
1 it protects mRNA from enzyme attack;
2 it is important in subsequent splicing;
3 it enhances translation of the mRNA.

The 5′ cap contains an 'inverted' base, 7-methylguanylate, attached to methylated ribose units.

The **3′ polyA tail** of mRNA has an unknown function. It is not encoded by the gene and is added after cutting of the primary mRNA transcript at the cleavage signal AAUAAA, which is recognized by a specific **endonuclease enzyme**. The polyA tail is not required for transcription, and some species of mRNA do not have a polyA tail.

SPLICING

Splicing is the removal of part, if not most, of the newly synthesized mRNA precursors. Only the mRNA corresponding to DNA **exons** are needed for transcription. Exons are the regions within the eukaryotic genes that are expressed, and in the DNA are separated from each other by **introns**, which are non-coding regions of the DNA. mRNA corresponding to the DNA introns is cut away from the pre-mRNA by specific splicing enzymes. All eukaryotic systems described so far have introns that begin with **5′-GU** and end with **AG-3′**. Eukaryotic DNA contains many non-coding regions of repetitious DNA, which has been called 'junk DNA'.

The **site** of splicing is determined by the 5′ and 3′ **splice sites** and a region of the intron called the **branch site**. The branch site is a short sequence of ribonucleotides which may vary with the cell type and the species. All three splice sites, i.e. 5′, 3′ and the branch site, must be in order for correct splicing. Mutations of the sites can cause disease due to incorrect splicing.

The mechanism of splicing requires: (i) the cutting of the 5′ splice site; (ii) the cutting of the 3′ splice site; (iii) the release of the intron in 'lariat' form (so-called because it resembles the cowboys' lasso); and (iv) the joining of the two exons which are on either side of the spliced intron. The two exons are joined by means of two **transesterification** reactions, in which the free –OH group of one exon is linked to the free 5′ phosphate of the other. While these steps are being carried out, the whole assembly is held together by the splicosome.

The **splicosome** is a relatively large 60S complex made up of the mRNA precursor and three different species of small nuclear RNA (snRNA). Molecules of snRNA have been nicknamed 'snurps' (small cytoplasmic RNA has been nicknamed 'scurps'). Different snurps have different functions in splicing.

Snurp (snRNA)	Function in splicosome
U_1	Binds 5′ splice site
U_2	Binds branch site
U_3	Binds 3′ splice site
U_4–U_6	Assembles the splicosome

Catalytic RNA (self-splicing) was discovered in protozoa, in which rRNA can splice itself in the absence of any protein, i.e. enzymes.

Catalytic RNA is stable, and appears to function like an enzyme. It has been shown to catalyse the cleavage and joining together of other nucleotides. It is therefore both a ribonuclease and an RNA polymerase. Furthermore, it exhibits the features of enzymes, being highly selective for substrates, obeying saturation kinetics and the kinetics of competitive inhibition. Self-splicing RNA is important evolutionarily, since biochemical reactions of DNA and RNA could have taken place even before the evolution of protein enzymes involved in DNA and RNA synthesis.

14 Errors of transcription

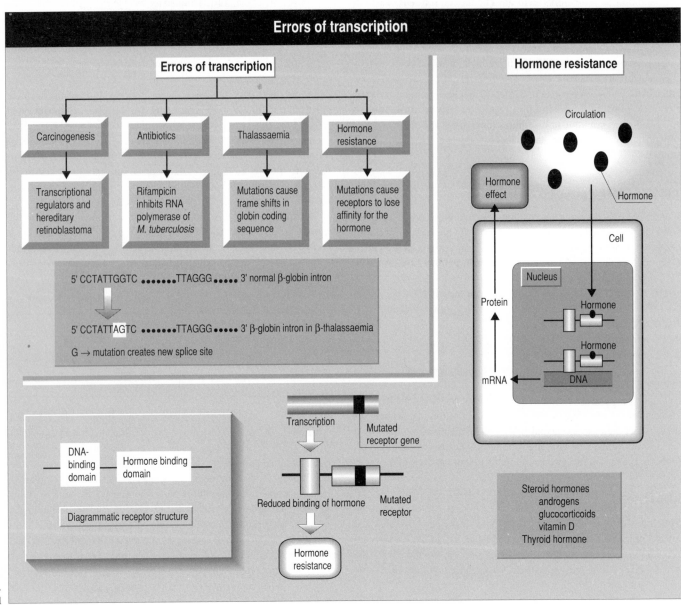

Errors of transcription

Errors of transcription

Carcinogenesis

Antibiotics

Thalassaemia

Hormone resistance

Transcriptional regulators and hereditary retinoblastoma

Rifampicin inhibits RNA polymerase of *M. tuberculosis*

Mutations cause frame shifts in globin coding sequence

Mutations cause receptors to lose affinity for the hormone

5' CCTATTGGTC ●●●●●●●TTAGGG ●●●●● 3' normal β-globin intron

5' CCTATTAGTC ●●●●●●●TTAGGG ●●●●● 3' β-globin intron in β-thalassaemia

G → mutation creates new splice site

DNA-binding domain

Hormone binding domain

Diagrammatic receptor structure

Transcription

Mutated receptor gene

Reduced binding of hormone

Mutated receptor

Hormone resistance

Hormone resistance

Circulation

Hormone effect

Hormone

Cell

Nucleus

Protein

Hormone

Hormone

mRNA

DNA

Steroid hormones
androgens
glucocorticoids
vitamin D
Thyroid hormone

Fig. 14.1

INTRODUCTION

Errors of transcription can result in disease, and transcription is vulnerable to toxic agents such as α-amanitin, and to certain antibiotics. Inappropriate expression of transcription and growth factors can cause cancer. Mutations of the DNA can cause changes in the location of splice sites, with resultant defective functional and structural proteins. These mutations can result in defective receptor proteins for hormones. The vulnerability of transcription to drugs such as fungal toxins and to antibiotics means that these are useful both as research tools and as potential chemotherapeutic agents.

CANCER

The conversion of normal cells into malignant cells is mediated by, for example, viruses, mutagenic chemicals and ionizing radiations. Malignant cells divide out of control and may kill the host organism if not stopped. Malignant cells may start producing their own growth factors and reduce or abolish their susceptibility to negative growth factors.

Transforming growth factors (TGFs) are chemicals that can convert a normal cell to a malignant cell. For example, there is evidence that the hormone progesterone increases the expression of a growth factor called TGF-α, which may mediate the growth of breast cancer cells. In another type of cancer, **hereditary retinoblastoma**, a rare cancer of the retina in infants, the cancer cells lack the **Rb gene**, which in normal cells may be a negative regulator of transcription.

ANTIBIOTICS

The antibiotic **rifampicin**, a semi-synthetic derivative of rifamycin, which was isolated from *Streptomyces*, blocks the formation of the first phosphodiester bond in RNA synthesis (see also p. 25). Chain elongation, however, is not affected. The bacterium that causes tuberculosis is *Mycobacterium tuberculosis*, and it is highly resistant to most antibiotics. But, it is susceptible to rifampicin, which is not as toxic to mammalian RNA polymerase. Rifampicin is used together with an antimetabolite, isoniazid, to treat the disease.

THALASSAEMIA

Thalassaemia (Cooley's anaemia) is an hereditary blood disease, especially prevalent in Africa, Asia and the Mediterranean countries, in which the globin part of the Hb molecule is altered, with decreased synthesis of the α- or β-chains. The geographical distribution of the disease coincides largely with that of malaria. Patients with the disease are anaemic because the Hb molecule cannot function normally. There are two types: (i) thalassaemia major, when the disease is inherited from both patients (i.e. there are two copies of the abnormal gene), and the patient is badly affected; and (ii) thalassaemia minor, when the defective gene is inherited from one parent, and the child has mild symptoms, or is free of symptoms. In thalassaemia major, affected individuals are anaemic and have swollen spleens and abnormalities of the bone marrow. They may require blood transfusions, which can result in an iron overload.

The disease can also be classified as **α-thalassaemia** or **β-thalassaemia**. α-Thalassaemia is a deficiency of the α-globin chains due to unequal crossover between adjacent α-alleles. β-Thalassaemia, which is rarer, can be due to one of a number of different mutations. For example, there is a G → A mutation of the β-globin coding region, resulting in a new splicing site; thus, a frame shift occurs. The promoter may be mutated, or the nascent mRNA prematurely released from the template strand or the splicing may be incorrect.

HORMONE RESISTANCE

Steroid and thyroid hormones, and vitamin D all act on their target cells by combining with intracellular receptors. The hormone–receptor complex binds to specific sequences upstream of transcription start sites and triggers transcription. The receptor protein has two important domains: one that binds the hormone and another that binds the DNA. This knowledge, and the knowledge of the structure of the genes that code for these receptors, has led to an understanding of the causes of several diseases characterized by a lack of responsiveness to these hormones.

For example, **androgen resistance** is the failure to respond to the male sex hormone testosterone, and to its powerful androgenic metabolite 5α-dihydrotestosterone (DHT). The disease may be caused by: (i) the complete or partial deletion of the gene that codes for the androgen receptor; (ii) splicing defects; (iii) premature termination codons; and (iv) amino acid substitutions resulting from mutated base substitutions. These mutations usually mean a loss of affinity of the hormone for the receptor. In the case of androgen resistance, most of the amino acid substitutions occur in the steroid-binding domain of the receptor.

Thyroid resistance, too, can be caused by mutations of the gene that codes for the thyroid receptor. These patients have retarded growth and lesions of bone, despite having high plasma levels of thyroid hormone. The tissues are not 'seeing' the hormone. Two distinct thyroid receptors, α and β, are encoded by two distinct genes, the α- and β-genes. In cases of generalized resistance to thyroid hormone, it has been discovered that most mutations occur within a tightly circumscribed region of the β-gene.

Glucocorticoid resistance can also be explained, in part, by mutations of the receptor, and this has important implications for therapy since glucocorticoids such as **prednisolone** are used extensively as anti-inflammatory agents in connective tissue diseases, and as immuno-suppressants in autoimmune diseases. Thus, patients who are resistant to glucocorticoids will not respond to treatment with them. In some cases of glucocorticoid resistance, **point mutations** have been discovered, resulting in the substitution of single amino acids. This results in a reduced affinity for the hormone.

15 Protein synthesis I

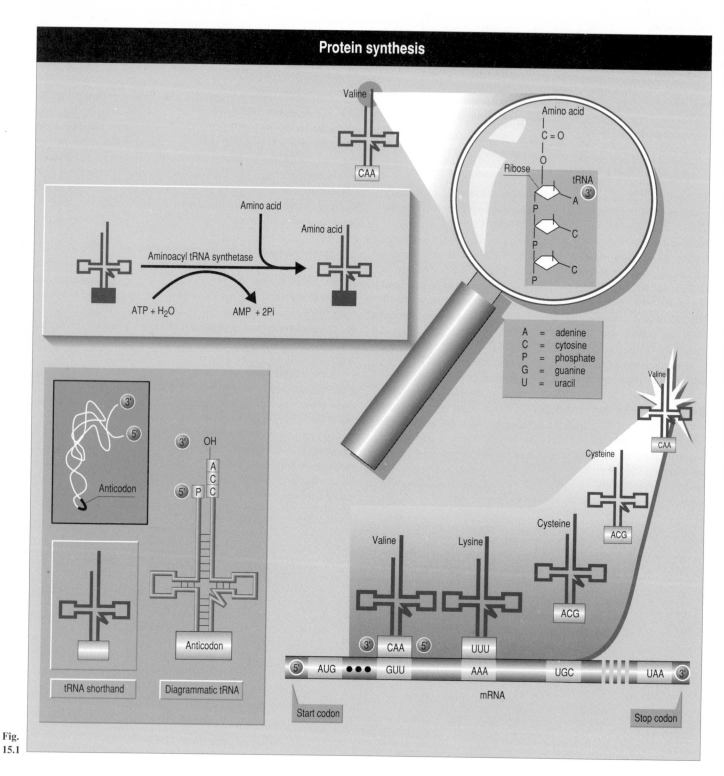

Fig. 15.1

INTRODUCTION

Proteins are synthesized by a process called **translation**. This is literally the translation of the sequence of bases in the DNA, and therefore in the corresponding mRNA, into a sequence of amino acids joined together to form the polypeptide chain, the primary structure of proteins. The primary structure will determine, in turn, the secondary and tertiary structure, and therefore the function of the protein. Protein synthesis, as in the case of DNA and RNA synthesis, takes place in three stages: (i) initiation; (ii) elongation; and (iii) termination. Amino acids are activated through linkage to their tRNA molecules in a reaction catalysed by an enzyme, an **aminoacyl–tRNA synthetase** specific for the particular amino acid. In some cases, there may be more than one tRNA and enzyme serving a particular amino acid. Polypeptide chains are elongated in the direction amino to carboxyl group ($NH_3^+ \rightarrow COO^-$), by the polysome 'assembly line'. An initiator tRNA triggers synthesis by binding to a site on the ribosome; elongation begins with the binding of another tRNA to another site; and termination occurs when a protein release factor 'reads' a stop signal on the mRNA.

THE GENETIC CODE

At least 20 different amino acids occur in proteins, but there are only four bases in DNA and mRNA, and it was discovered that a sequence of three bases, called a **codon**, codes for each amino acid. The number of possible triplet codons derived from four bases is $4^3 = 64$. Experiments have determined that of these, 61 combinations code for amino acids. Although some amino acids, for example tryptophan, have only one codon (UGG), others, for example serine, have as many as six (see below). Nevertheless, the genetic code is specific and unambiguous; one codon codes for one amino acid only.

5′ end of codon	Middle base of codon				3′ end of codon
	U	C	A	G	
U	Phe	Ser	Tyr	Cys	U
U	Phe	Ser	Tyr	Cys	C
U	Leu	Ser	STOP	STOP	A
U	Leu	Ser	STOP	Trp	G
C	Leu	Pro	His	Arg	U
C	Leu	Pro	His	Arg	C
C	Leu	Pro	Gln	Arg	A
C	Leu	Pro	Gln	Arg	G
A	Ile	Thr	Asn	Ser	U
A	Ile	Thr	Asn	Ser	C
A	Ile	Thr	Lys	Arg	A
A	Met*	Thr	Lys	Arg	G
G	Val	Ala	Asp	Gly	U
G	Val	Ala	Asp	Gly	C
G	Val	Ala	Glu	Gly	A
G	Val	Ala	Glu	Gly	G

* The codon for methionine (AUG) is a START codon for translation (see p. 30). For definitions of abbreviations see Abbreviations, p. 108.

Because there is more than one codon for amino acids, the code is referred to as **degenerate**. The code is also virtually **universal**, since substantially the same code has been found in all living organisms.

Codon	Mitochondrion	Normal meaning
CUA	Thr	Leu
AUA	Met	Ile
UGA	Trp	STOP

Mitochondria provide the only known exception to the rule of universality, since some codons which normally have one meaning are different in mitochondria.

The START signal for protein biosynthesis in eukaryotes is AUG, the codon for methionine. Methionine is therefore the first amino acid of the protein chain. The STOP signals, UGA, UAA and UAG, do not code for any amino acids, and may sometimes be referred to as **nonsense codons**.

THE 'WOBBLE' HYPOTHESIS

The 'wobble' hypothesis is an explanation for the fact that: (i) one tRNA can read more than one codon; and (ii) many of the codons can be read by more than one species of tRNA. Note, however, that one tRNA can carry only one species of amino acid; (i) and (ii) may be possible because the stringency requirements for base pairing normally stipulated by the Crick–Watson base-pairing rule do not apply, allowing base pairing between the third position of the codon on the mRNA reading $5' \rightarrow 3'$, and the first position of anticodon on the tRNA $5' \rightarrow 3'$. This makes the nucleotides literally wobble, changing the geometry of the codon–anticodon interaction, and allowing G–U base pairs to form. Wobble, and therefore the relaxation of stringency of base pairing between anticodon and codon in protein synthesis, may also be induced by the presence of modified nucleotides at or near the first position of the anticodon in some tRNA species. An important modified nucleotide for wobble is **inosinic acid** (I), which can form base pairs with A, C or U in the third position of mRNA codon. The relaxation of stringency of the base-pairing rule during wobble means that, theoretically, many of the different codons could be read by relatively few tRNA anticodons. In nature, however, this possibility has not necessarily been exploited, since most cells contain almost as many species of tRNA as there are of amino acids.

THE AMINOACYLATION REACTION

Amino acids are activated for protein synthesis, i.e. raised to a higher energy level for participation in protein synthesis, through coupling to tRNA in a reaction catalysed by a specific **aminoacyl–tRNA synthetase**. There are 20 different enzymes; one for each amino acid. The enzyme can: (i) recognize its specific amino acid–tRNA complex; and (ii) proofread the complex after it has bound it, and hydrolyse the incorrectly bound complex. It is not known with certainty how the enzyme proofreads the complex.

16 Protein synthesis II

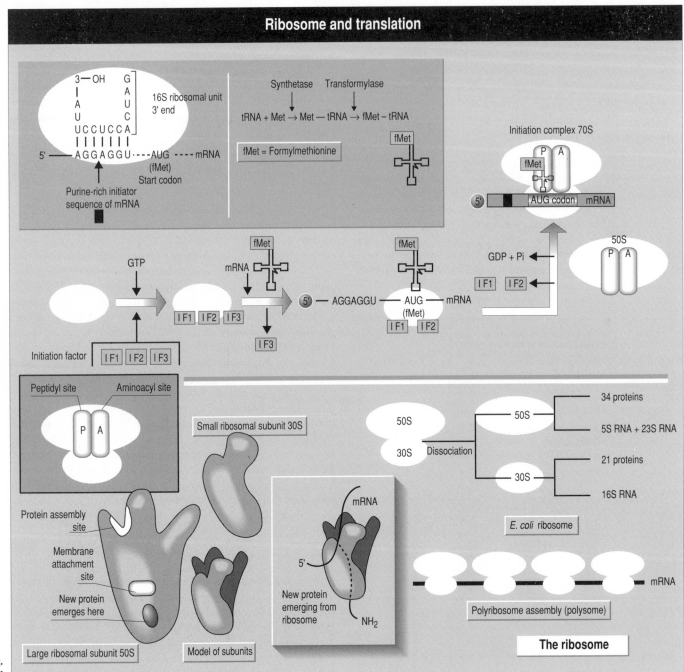

Ribosome and translation

Synthetase   Transformylase

tRNA + Met → Met — tRNA → fMet – tRNA

fMet = Formylmethionine

16S ribosomal unit 3' end

Purine-rich initiator sequence of mRNA

5' — AGGAGGU ···· AUG ···· mRNA
(fMet)
Start codon

Initiation complex 70S

Initiation factor

Peptidyl site   Aminoacyl site

Protein assembly site

Membrane attachment site

New protein emerges here

Large ribosomal subunit 50S

Small ribosomal subunit 30S

Model of subunits

New protein emerging from ribosome

Dissociation

34 proteins
5S RNA + 23S RNA
21 proteins
16S RNA

E. coli ribosome

Polyribosome assembly (polysome)

The ribosome

Fig. 16.1

INTRODUCTION

Protein synthesis is effected by the **ribosomes**, which are ribonucleoprotein particles. Ribosomes consist of two main subunits which fit together to form a structure that coordinates the assembly of proteins.

THE RIBOSOME

Bacterial ribosomes

In bacteria such as *E. coli*, whose ribosome has been extensively studied, the ribosome is an irregularly shaped ribonucleoprotein particle having a sedimentation coefficient of 70S, a diameter of about

20 nm and a mass of approximately 2700 kDa. The ribosome can be **dissociated** in the laboratory into a large 50S subunit and a smaller 30S subunit. These subunits can be dissociated further into the proteins and rRNA which make them up. The structure and function of the ribosome depends principally on the way the constituent rRNA molecules fold and associate with the proteins. Each bacterial cell has about 20 000 ribosomes, which constitute roughly 25% of the mass of the cell. Viewed under the electron microscope, ribosomes may be observed free in the cytoplasm.

Eukaryotic ribosomes

In mammalian cells, the structure and function of the ribosome is very similar to that of the *E. coli* ribosome, although its composition differs. The mammalian ribosome is 80S, having a mass of 42 kDa, and dissociates into 60S and 40S subunits. The 40S subunit has an 18S rRNA molecule and about 30 associated proteins, and the 40S subunit is made up of 5S, 5.8S and 28S rRNA, and about 45 associated proteins. Viewed under the electron microscope, ribosomes may be observed free in the cytoplasm or firmly attached to the ER. As a general rule, free ribosomes synthesize proteins for use in the cytoplasm, while membrane-bound ribosomes synthesize proteins for export from the cell, or for making membranes.

TRANSLATION

For protein synthesis, several ribosomes can bind simultaneoulsy to a mRNA molecule to form a polyribosome, or **polysome**. There may be up to one ribosome attached every eight nucleotides along the mRNA. The individual ribosomes of the polysome work independently of each other, and each produces a complete polypeptide chain. Polypeptide chains are synthesized in the direction $NH_2 \rightarrow COOH$, and the mRNA is read from 5' to 3'. In eukaryotes, mRNA is exported from the nucleus to the cytoplasm, where protein synthesis occurs, whereas in prokaryotes such as *E. coli*, a mRNA molecule may be translated even while it is being transcribed.

Initiation in prokaryotes

Protein synthesis in prokaryotic cells is initiated by the combination, in the cytosol (see p. 30), of the free, smaller subunit of the ribosome with an initiator **tRNA** molecule that carries the amino acid methionine (Met). The initiator tRNA: (i) is linked with Met through a reaction catalysed by the corresponding aminoacyl–tRNA synthetase; and (ii) the Met attached to the tRNA is formylated by a transformylase ('formyl' is derived from formic acid, HCOOH). The initiator tRNA is therefore expressed as tRNA$_f$. The Met attached to tRNA$_f$ does not usually form part of the final polypeptide chain, but is removed after the protein has been made.

> *Note*: Met attached to an intiator tRNA$_f$ can be formylated, but it cannot be formylated if attached to the species of tRNA that carries a molecule of Met destined for permanent inclusion in the protein. In this latter case, the tRNA that carries Met is designated tRNA$_{Met}$, or tRNA$_m$.

The free, smaller 30S subunit binds three initiation factors (IFs), IF1, IF2 and IF3. IF2 binds GTP, and also recognizes the Met–tRNA$_f$ complex. The reaction between IF2 and GTP also enables the mRNA molecule to be bound by the 30S subunit. IF3 dissociates as the 30S–Met–tRNA$_f$ complex is formed; GTP is hydrolysed as the larger 50S subunit joins the complex; and IF1 and IF2 dissociate. The Met–tRNA$_f$ molecule is located in the **P site** of the ribosome, and the **A site** is empty at the start of the elongation phase of protein synthesis. The resultant 70S complex is termed the **initiation complex.**

The Shine–Dalgarno sequence

The Met–tRNA$_f$ molecule has the anticodon UAC, which binds non-covalently to the initiation codon AUG on the mRNA molecule. AUG codes for Met. In *E. coli*, the site of initiation is situated at a purine-rich region of the mRNA upstream from the AUG start codon, and this purine-rich region is called the **Shine–Dalgarno** sequence (e.g. for *E. coli lacI*, the sequence is 5'-AGGAGG-3'). This sequence pairs with a complementary sequence very near the 3' end of the 16S rRNA of the 30S subunit.

Therefore, protein synthesis will be initiated where the anticodon of the tRNA$_f$ binds the initiator AUG codon, and where the mRNA pairs with the complementary sequence at the 3' end of the 16S rRNA molecule.

Initiation in eukaryotes

The mechanism of initiation of translation in eukaryotic cells is fundamentally the same as in prokaryotes, but with some differences.
1 The initiating tRNA is Met and **not** formylmethionine (fMet). The tRNA carrying Met is termed tRNA$_i$.
2 There are many more IFs (at least nine are known, and doubtless more will be discovered):
   (a) eIF2 binds GTP and escorts tRNA to the 40S complex;
   (b) cap-binding proteins bind to the mRNA 5' cap, and eIF3 binds to the AUG start codon nearest to the cap, using energy provided by eIF4, which in turn derives its energy from ATP;
   (c) Met–tRNA$_i$ binds to the start codon AUG and eIF5 causes eIF2 to hydrolyse GTP, which results in the release of eIF2 and eIF3 from the initiation complex;
   (d) the 60S subunit is attached to form the complete initiation complex.

> *Note*: in eukaryotes, there is one start codon only — AUG — and no Shine–Dalgarno purine-rich sequence. The 40S complex attaches itself to the mRNA at the 5' end and uses energy (ATP see (2a) above) to move towards the 3' end until it finds the AUG start signal.

17 Protein synthesis III

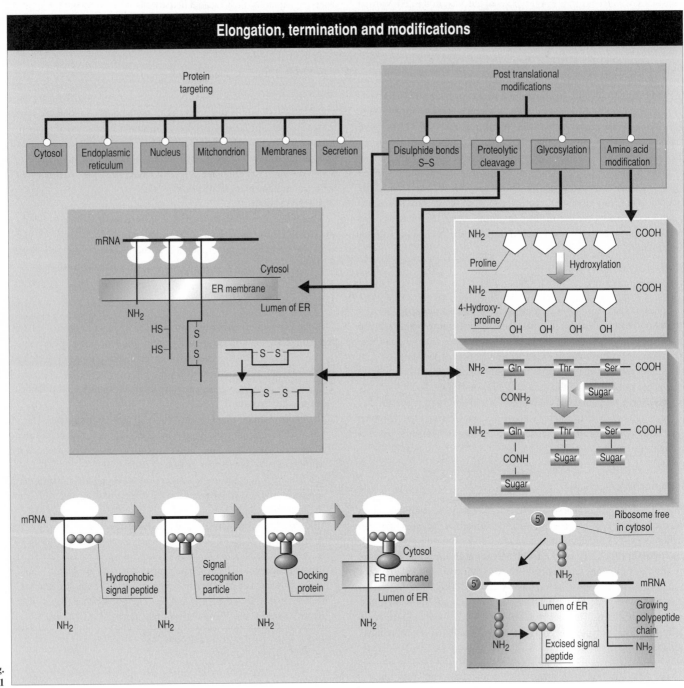

Fig. 17.1

INTRODUCTION

After the initiation of protein synthesis, the peptide chain is elongated, and when the appropriate signal is reached, elongation is terminated. The peptide is released from the ribosomal apparatus, and may be subject to post-translational modification. The protein will be modified depending on whether it is destined for other cellular organelles, such as mitochondria, the nucleus or lysosomes, or to structural units, such as the cell membrane. It may be modified for export. Errors in post-translational modification may result in disease.

ELONGATION

The amino acid to be added to the initial methionine is delivered, attached to its tRNA, to the A site of the ribosome by an **elongation factor**. It is critically important that the correct aminoacyl–tRNA is in the A site, because the cell cannot excise a 'wrong' amino acid once it has been added to the chain. The 'proofreading' is done by an elongation factor, **EF-TU** in prokaryotes. EF-TU binds GTP, and this enables it to bind the aminoacyl–tRNA and bring it to the A site. The amino acid cannot be added to the chain until EF-TU leaves the complex, and EF-TU cannot leave until it has hydrolysed its GTP to GDP. Therefore, there is time, while GTP is being hydrolysed, and while the EF-TU is leaving the complex, for an incorrect aminoacyl–tRNA to leave the complex. In eukaryotes, the proofreading elongation factor is **EF1**, whose subunit EF1α forms a complex with the aminoacyl–tRNA.

Elongation has two main steps, **peptide bond formation** and **translocation**. Peptide bond formation is catalysed by peptidyl transferase, which attaches the carbonyl atom of the P site aminoacyl–tRNA to the α-amino group of the amino acid of the aminoacyl–tRNA in the A site. The A site must now be emptied for the next aminoacyl–tRNA, and so the reading frame is shifted three bases along the mRNA until the next codon is at the A site. This movement is driven by another elongation factor, or **translocase**, which utilizes GTP hydrolysis for energy. In prokaryotes, the factor is EF-G, and in eukaryotes it is **EF2**. During the process, the tRNA–OH whose amino acid has been removed is shifted to a so-called 'exit site' on the ribosome, from where it is released back into the cytoplasm. In eukaryotes, a number of other elongation factors have been identified but their exact roles are not clear.

Termination

When a termination or STOP codon is reached, no aminoacyl–tRNA can be accepted in the A site. Instead, the codon is bound by a release factor–GTP complex **RF–GTP**. As a result, peptidyl transferase switches to being a hydrolase, adding H_2O to the carbonyl end of the peptide chain. RF hydrolyses its GTP to GDP, and undergoes a conformational change. These changes provide the energy to dissociate the elongation complex into the constituent mRNA, polypeptide chain and the ribosomal subunits. In prokaryotes, three release factors have been described: RF1, RF2 and RF3. RF1 and RF2 recognize different STOP codons, and RF3 potentiates the actions of RF1 and RF2.

Prokaryote–eukaryote protein synthesis summary

Feature	Prokaryotes	Eukaryotes
Large ribosome subunit	50S	60S
Small ribosome subunit	30S	40S
Whole ribosome	70S	80S
Large subunit rRNA	5S 23S	5S 5.8S 28S
Small subunit RNA	16S	18S
Large subunit protein numbers	34 proteins	50 proteins
Small subunit protein numbers	21 proteins	34 proteins
Initiation factors	IF1 IF2 IF3	eIF2 eIF3 eIF4a eIF4b eIF4c eIF5 eIF6 cap-binding protein
Initiating aminoacyl–tRNA	fMet–tRNA	Met–tRNA
Pre-start purine-rich sequence	Shine–Dalgarno	None
Elongation factors	EF-G (translocase)	EF1 EF2 (translocase)
Release factors	RF1 RF2 RF3	RF

Post-translational modifications

The amino acid sequence and conformational shape of a protein will determine its fate, whether it is to be targeted to a particular site, or to be a substrate for modifying enzymes. They will also determine its half-life.

Eukaryote ribosomes that produce lysosomal proteins, membrane proteins and proteins for export are bound to the ER. During protein synthesis in the cytosol, a **signal sequence** rich in hydrophobic residues, such as phenylalanine, is produced near the amino terminus. The sequence is recognized by a ribonucleoprotein termed **signal recognition particle (SRP)**, which binds to the ribosome, enabling it to bind to the surface of the ER at a 'docking' protein called **SRP receptor**. The ribosome interlocks with two ER membrane translocation proteins called **Riophorin I** and **II**, which drive the elongating peptide chain through the ER membrane into the lumen of the ER. Once inside the lumen, the signal sequence is excised.

Inside the lumen of the ER, several modifications may occur: (i) the protein may be crosslinked by disulphide bonds; (ii) part of the chain may be excised by proteolysis, for example the removal of an inactive portion of several prohormones, such as the conversion of proinsulin to insulin, for export; and (iii) proteins may be glycosylated. Glycosylation of proteins serves three main purposes: (i) changes their physical properties, for example solubility, size and stability; (ii) the carbohydrate addition is an important component of a membrane protein which has to recognize other proteins or cells; and (iii) enables the protein to be targeted to specific cellular sites.

In the lumen, oligosaccharides may be carried to the growing peptide chain by a lipid carrier, **dolichol phosphate**, which is located on the luminal surface of the ER membrane. The oligosaccharide attached to the dolichol phosphate becomes attached to an asparagine (Asn) residue on the peptide, in a reaction catalysed by a **glycosyltransferase**. Glycosylation may take place after the protein has moved through the ER to the **Golgi apparatus**, where it may also be packaged into vesicles for exocytosis if it is for export.

Proteins may be modified during translation (cotranslationally) through the alteration of amino acids. For example, in collagen synthesis, proline is hydroxylated to hydroxyproline.

TARGETING

To the mitochondrion

Proteins targeted to specific cellular sites need special signals. Most proteins destined for the mitochondrion are released into the cytoplasm by free ribosomes, and their signal will differ depending on whether they are targeted to the mitochondrial membranes or to the mitochondrial matrix. Once inside the mitochondrion, the targeting signal is usually cleaved from the protein.

To the nucleus

Most proteins destined for the cell nucleus have specific signal sequences rich in arginine and lysine sequences. The localization of histones to the nucleus appears to be mediated by a protein termed **nucleoplasmin**.

'Proofreading' aminoacyl–tRNA in A site of ribosome

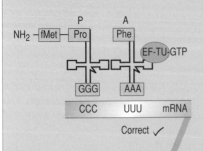

CCC — UUU — mRNA

Correct ✓

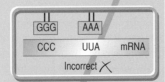

CCC — UUA — mRNA

Incorrect ✗

NH₂ – fMet – Pro / Phe   EF-TU·GDP + Pi

GGG — AAA

CCC — UUU — mRNA

Correct ✓

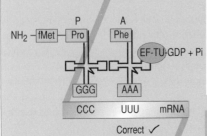

CCC — UUA — mRNA

Incorrect ✗

EF-TU·GDP + Pi ←

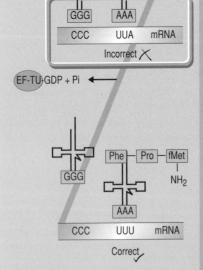

CCC — UUU — mRNA

Correct ✓

Termination

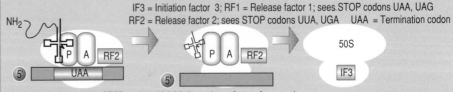

IF3 = Initiation factor 3; RF1 = Release factor 1; sees STOP codons UAA, UAG
RF2 = Release factor 2; sees STOP codons UUA, UGA   UAA = Termination codon

50S

IF3

Termination occurs with a STOP codon which binds a release factor. As a result
(i) Peptidyl transferase forms a COOH terminus to the polypeptide, which dissociates
(ii) tRNA and mRNA dissociate from the complex
(iii) The ribosome dissociates into 50S and 30S subunits. IF3 binds to 30S and prevents premature binding of 30S and 50S.

Peptide bond formation

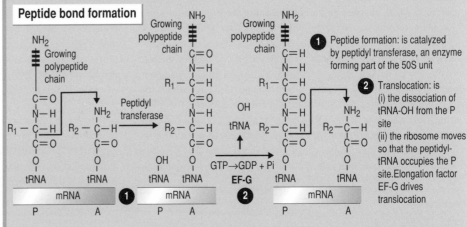

❶ Peptide formation: is catalyzed by peptidyl transferase, an enzyme forming part of the 50S unit

❷ Translocation: is
(i) the dissociation of tRNA-OH from the P site
(ii) the ribosome moves so that the peptidyl-tRNA occupies the P site. Elongation factor EF-G drives translocation

Elongation factor cycle

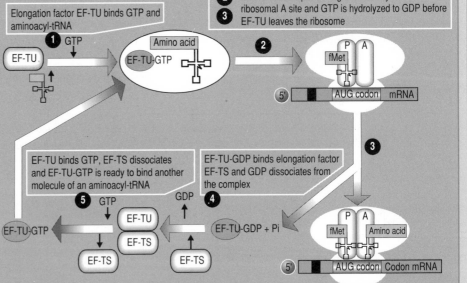

Elongation factor EF-TU binds GTP and aminoacyl-tRNA

❷ EF-TU enables positioning of aminoacyl-tRNA in
❸ ribosomal A site and GTP is hydrolyzed to GDP before EF-TU leaves the ribosome

EF-TU binds GTP, EF-TS dissociates and EF-TU-GTP is ready to bind another molecule of an aminoacyl-tRNA

EF-TU-GDP binds elongation factor EF-TS and GDP dissociates from the complex

Fig.
17.2

PATHOPHYSIOLOGY OF PROTEIN MODIFICATION

Several diseases and abnormal protein status situations arise from errors in the post-translational modification of proteins, including errors in the targeting process.

Familial hyperproinsulinaemia is an autosomal dominant state in which the individual has approximately the same amount of proinsulin and insulin in the circulation. Those with the condition may exhibit none of the symptoms of diabetes, and glucose metabolism is apparently normal, despite the presence of very high levels of proinsulin in the blood. The cause of the condition is not known with certainty, but may involve point mutations in the proinsulin molecule, which prevents the action of the protease enzymes which splice proinsulin.

I-cell disease is one of a number of related disorders arising from aberrations in the targeting of lysosomal enzymes. Other diseases are **mucolipidosis II** and **III**. The lesion is a deficiency in the enzyme which catalyses the transfer of *N*-acetylglucosamine phosphate to polysaccharide moieties of proteins which are targeted to the lysosome. These proteins are secreted into the bloodstream, and are found in high concentrations in a number of body fluids. The defect is usually present at birth and manifested by skeletal abnormalities, facial coarsening of features and psychomotor retardation. Patients usually die before 7–8 years of age.

18 Errors of translation

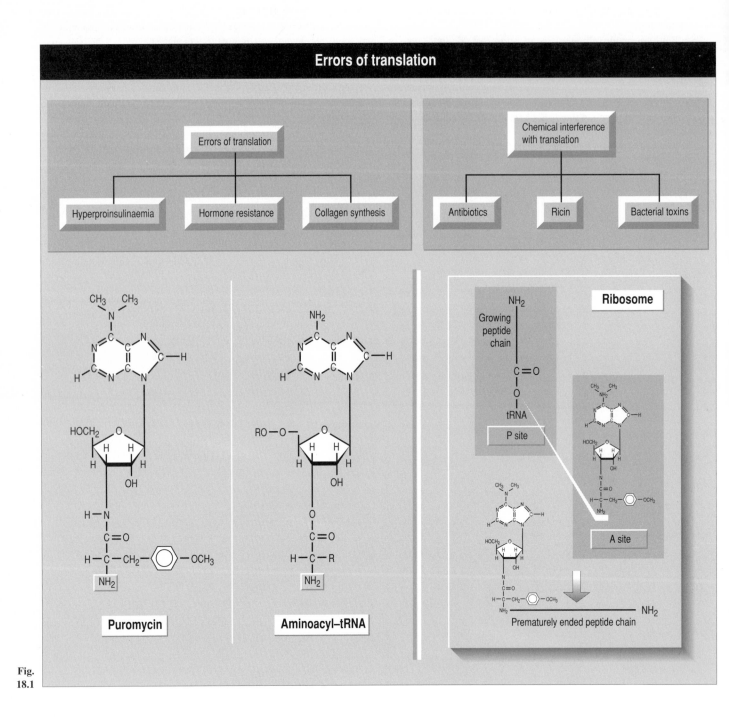

Errors of translation

Errors of translation
- Hyperproinsulinaemia
- Hormone resistance
- Collagen synthesis

Chemical interference with translation
- Antibiotics
- Ricin
- Bacterial toxins

Puromycin

Aminoacyl–tRNA

Ribosome

NH₂
Growing peptide chain
C=O
O
tRNA
P site

A site

Prematurely ended peptide chain

Fig. 18.1

Protein synthesis can be blocked by drugs, termed **antibiotics**. This term encompasses agents that have actions other than translation. They may interfere with cell wall synthesis or with intermediary metabolism. They are useful tools for elucidating the mechanisms of translation, and some are extremely useful therapeutically because they target the prokaryote translation machinery specifically. Defects in the translation process may also be responsible for several diseases in humans.

INHIBITORS OF PROTEIN SYNTHESIS

Antibiotics

Streptomycin and **neomycin** are aminoglycoside antibiotics extensively used therapeutically. Streptomycin inhibits initiation by binding to the 30S ribosomal subunit and interfering with the functioning of a single ribosomal protein called S12, which mediates the binding of

Inhibitor	Site of inhibition	Process inhibited
Chloramphenicol	Prokaryote 50S subunit	Peptidyl transferase
Cycloheximide	Eukaryote 80S ribosome	Elongation
Erythromycin	Prokaryote 50S subunit	Translocation
Fusidic acid	Prokaryote EF-G action	Translocation
Neomycins	Prokaryotes many sites	Translation
Puromycin*	Ribosome	Peptide transfer
Ricin	Eukaryote	Many processes
Streptomycin	Prokaryote 30S subunit	Initiation Elongation
Tetracyclines	Prokaryote 30S subunit	Aminoacyl–tRNA Binding

* Eukaryotes and prokaryotes.

fMet–aminoacyl–tRNA and mRNA to the ribosome. It also causes misreading of the mRNA codons. Neomycin does not appear to act through S12. **Tetracyclines** also bind to the ribosome and block aminoacyl–tRNA binding. They were heavily prescribed in children until it was discovered that they stained their permanent teeth yellow. **Chloramphenicol** is toxic to a wide variety of microorganisms, but is also seriously toxic to bone marrow, and is reserved for dangerous diseases such as typhoid fever, or for localized (topical) application in, for example eye drops.

Antibiotics, such as **cycloheximide** and **puromycin**, which attack both prokaryotic and eukaryotic translation, are virtually useless therapeutically, but are very powerful experimental tools. Puromycin resembles the terminal aminoacyl–adenosine part of the aminoacyl–tRNA and therefore competes with it for the binding site on the A site of the ribosome. Puromycin becomes incorporated into the growing peptide chain at the carboxyl end because it has an α-amino group recognized by peptidyl transferase. **Ricin** is a plant toxin from castor beans, that has N-glycosidase activity and attacks the ribosome directly, cleaving an adenine base from the large subunit. Recently, in Spain, many hundreds of people died after using cooking oil contaminated with ricin.

Translation can also be inhibited by **bacterial toxins**. For example, a protein toxin produced by the diphtheria-producing bacterium *Corynebacterium diphtheria*, enzymatically inactivates EF2 by converting it to ADP–ribosyl EF2.

TRANSLATION AND DISEASE

Several, usually familial, diseases are caused by defects in the translation process. These may involve alterations to the **cleavage** of newly synthesized peptide chains, or defects in the **targeting** of proteins or from **mutations** in the genes, and thus in the mRNA, resulting in the incorporation of the wrong amino acid into the protein.

Cleavage

Defects of cleavage are responsible for **familial hyperproinsulinaemia**, in which affected individuals have abnormally high circulating levels of the insulin precursor proinsulin. Normally, the insulin gene codes for a large precursor, preproinsulin, which is released into the lumen of the ER. The signal sequence is cleaved by a signal peptidase to yield a smaller protein, proinsulin. This is transported to the Golgi apparatus, where it is packaged into vesicles for export. Inside the vesicle, the molecule is cleaved further to remove the so-called C peptide, an internal peptide chain, and bioactive insulin is eventually released by exocytosis.

Receptor defects and hormone resistance

Errors of translation can result in **hormone resistance**. This is a failure of the target cell to respond to certain hormones, for example androgens, glucocorticoids, thyroid hormones and vitamin D, which all act through intracellular receptors

In patients with **androgen** resistance, these receptors may be: (i) absent altogether; (ii) grossly altered in structure due to deletion of segments of the carboxyterminal end of the polypeptide chain; or (iii) altered in just one amino acid (a **point mutation**, which results from a mutation of a single base pair in the DNA). All these are due to mutations of the androgen receptor gene, and the condition is therefore familial. As a result, the patient does not respond to his own androgen, and is infertile.

Mutations of different regions of the **low-density lipoprotein (LDL) receptor gene** can cause a disruption of cholesterol metabolism, and lead to hypercholesterolaemia and premature vascular disease. The mutation may result in: (i) a reduced number of receptors or none at all; (ii) a reduced rate of transport of the newly synthesized receptor from the ER to the Golgi apparatus; (iii) the failure of the LDL receptor to bind LDL; or (iv) failure of recycling of LDL receptors. These diseases are usually familial.

There are defects of translation of the proteins of **collagen**, resulting in structural weaknesses of collagen, an important supporting tissue in the body.

19 Collagen

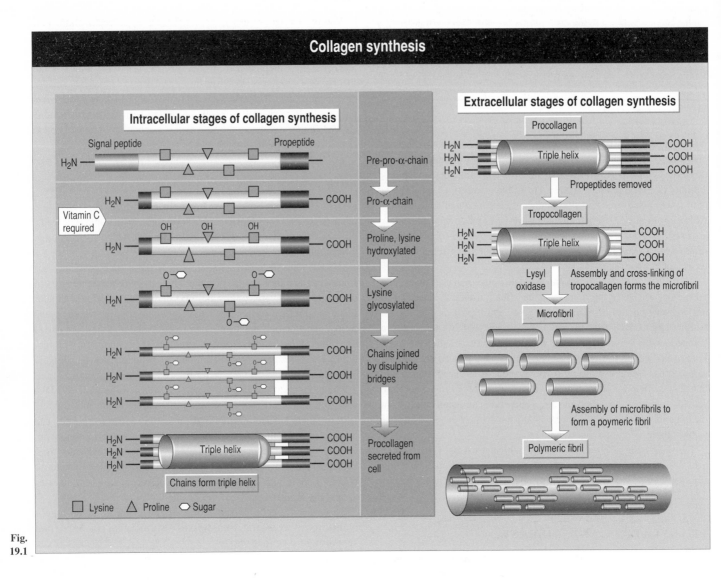

Collagen synthesis

Intracellular stages of collagen synthesis

Signal peptide — Propeptide

Pre-pro-α-chain

Vitamin C required

Pro-α-chain

Proline, lysine hydroxylated

Lysine glycosylated

Chains joined by disulphide bridges

Triple helix

Chains form triple helix

Procollagen secreted from cell

☐ Lysine △ Proline ⬡ Sugar

Extracellular stages of collagen synthesis

Procollagen

Triple helix

Propeptides removed

Tropocollagen

Triple helix

Lysyl oxidase — Assembly and cross-linking of tropocallagen forms the microfibril

Microfibril

Assembly of microfibrils to form a poymeric fibril

Polymeric fibril

Fig. 19.1

Collagen is used in this chapter as an example of the events in protein synthesis described in previous chapters.

NATURE OF COLLAGEN

Occurrence and structure

Collagen is a fibrous, secretory protein, the most abundant protein in the human body, and occurs in all tissues that demand a framework or support in order to give them structural strength and retention of their characteristic shape or form. Other examples of fibrous proteins are tropomyosin and α-keratin. Structurally, fibrous proteins possess a high proportion of regular secondary structure and a rod-like cylindrical shape, and are relatively insoluble in H_2O.

Each collagen peptide, referred to as an α-chain, occurs as a left-handed helical polypeptide, in which every third residue is a glycine, and is about 1000 residues long. Three α-chains intertwine to form a right-handed triple helix, and the glycine residues are at the centre of the helix. This helical structure is termed **tropocollagen**, and it is the fundamental building block or repeating unit of collagen.

Tropocollagen

Tropocollagen can be expressed in terms of an approximate structural formula: $(Gly–A–B)_{333}$, where proline occupies approximately one-third of the A positions, and about one-third of the B positions are occupied by hydroxyproline. Tropocollagen molecules spontaneously combine through a crosslinking between lysine and hydroxylysine residues, to form the so-called polymeric fibrils, which can be seen under the electron microscope, and these aggregate to form the light microscope-visible polymeric collagen fibres.

The rigidity of collagen is due to the presence of proline residues. The strength of collagen is provided by the fact that tropocollagen molecules are adjacent to each other along approximately 75% of the length of each molecule. Because of the way they are attached, they also resist stretching, or tensing, and will rupture if subjected to excessive tensile forces.

Types of collagen

Different tissues possess different types of collagen, of which there are at least 13, called type I, II, etc., up to XIII. Collagen types differ in terms of the α-chains, which are termed α1 and α2. Type I, the first to be characterized, is present in the largest abundance in the human body.

SYNTHESIS OF COLLAGEN

Collagen is synthesized by several different specialized cell types, for example by the osteoblasts in bone, fibroblasts in the tendons and by chondroblasts in cartilage. Synthesis may be thought of in terms of intracellular and extracellular events.

Intracellular events

In the cell, the first step is the synthesis of an α-chain by the ER-attached ribosomes, which translate the α-chain sequence from the mRNA as well as the propeptide sequences, and the N-terminal signal peptide, which directs the newly formed protein into the lumen of the ER. The propeptide sequences ensure that the precursors remain soluble, as they do not form a helix. In the lumen, the enzyme signal peptidase removes the signal sequence, and the pro-α-chain moves along the smooth ER and the Golgi apparatus towards the plasma membrane.

During this voyage, –OH groups are added to proline and lysyl residues which use **vitamin C** as a cofactor. The sugar residues glucose and galactose are added to hydroxylysine; the extent of glycosylation determining the thickness of the resultant collagen fibrils. The sugar residues reduce the degree of packing of the tropocollagen microfibrils into polymeric fibrils. The extent of the glycosylation depends on the tissue in which collagen is formed.

During the late stages of glycosylation, three pro-α-chains are formed into a unit by thiol (SH) bonds between the propeptides at the C terminal, and the linked chains coil into the characteristic triple helix of tropocollagen. The Golgi apparatus packages the soluble precursor (procollagen) into vesicles, which are secreted from the cell by pinocytosis.

Extracellular events

Once outside the cell, the fibre-forming collagens (types I, II and III) lose the propeptides by enzymatic cleavage to yield tropocollagen. (Type IV tropocollagen does not lose the propeptides.) These molecules spontaneously aggregate to form fibrils, and as the polypeptide chains build up a network of crosslinkages, so the strength of the collagen fibres increases.

PATHOPHYSIOLOGY

Scurvy

Scurvy is the result of a deficiency of vitamin C (ascorbic acid), whose lack in the diet causes a decrease in the synthesis of hydroxyproline. (Note, unlike many other animals, humans lack the enzymes required to synthesize ascorbic acid from glucose.) Hydroxyproline contributes additional hydrogen bonding for stabilization of collagen helices. As a result, collagen loses its stability at body temperature, and structures cannot adhere to connective tissues. The consequences include suppression of growth in children, capillary fragility and delayed and deficient wound healing. Teeth become dislodged from the gums, and sudden death can result in extreme cases if the patient changes posture.

Other disorders

There are, in addition, a number of genetic disorders that result in:
1 failure of collagen fibrils to crosslink, for example, **osteogenesis imperfecta**, where point mutations in the α-chain prevent helix formation, and enzymatic destruction of the tropocollagen molecules occurs; and
2 deficiency of certain enzymes, such as lysylhydroxylase, which is called **Ehlers–Danlos syndrome type VI**. Here, synthesis of hydroxylysine is suppressed.

These diseases are characterized by poor wound healing, multiple fractures and hyperextensible skin and joints.

20 Control of gene expression in prokaryotes

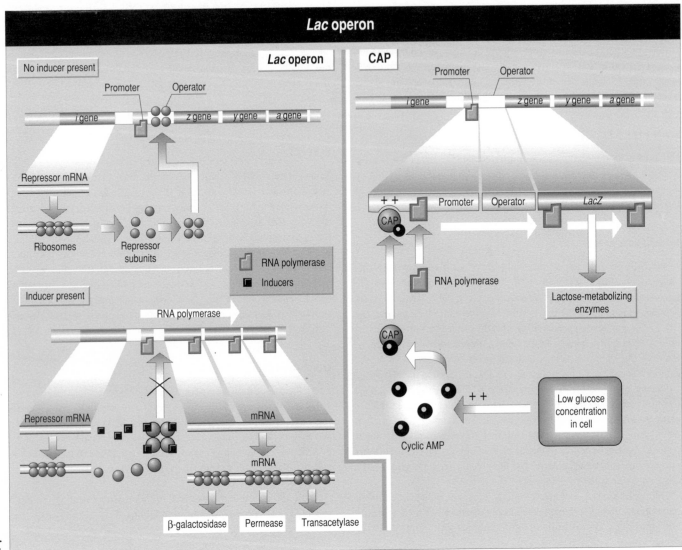

Fig. 20.1

PROKARYOTES

E. coli is a bacterium in which gene expression has been extensively studied and characterized. *E. coli* has a single, circular chromosome, composed of a double-stranded DNA molecule of about 4×10^6 base pairs. There are about 3000 genes, which are clustered according to function. For example, the genes coding for enzymes of a particular metabolic pathway are clustered, as are those coding for structural proteins. These clustered genes are usually under co-ordinate control, and are transcribed together to form a single strand of mRNA that codes for several different proteins. Such an mRNA strand is termed **polycistronic mRNA**, and a complete set of functionally clustered genes, together with their operator and regulatory genes, is termed an **operon**.

Regulatory genes code for proteins that in turn control expression of

the genes by binding to **control elements** at sites on the DNA near to the structural gene. Regulatory proteins control the degree of access that the enzyme **RNA polymerase** has to its binding site on the gene. Two types of regulatory protein have been found: (i) negatively acting, which repress the operon by binding to the operator; and (ii) positively acting, which enhance the affinity of RNA polymerase for its binding sites on the gene. A good example of an operon is the lactose operon of *E. coli*.

THE LACTOSE OPERON

Expression of the operon is regulated by an **inducer** (lactose), and by a **repressor protein**, expressed by the *i* gene. The *i* gene (also called *lacI*), is situated just before the controlling elements for the cluster of genes coding for three enzymes, at least two of which are important in the splitting of the disaccharide lactose into galactose and glucose. These three genes, called the *lacZYA* cluster, code for: (i) **β-galactosidase**, which acts on lactose; (ii) **β-galactoside permease**, a membrane-bound protein which forms part of the transport system for taking lactose into the cell; and (iii) **β-galactoside transacetylase**, whose precise function is unknown, but whose expression is essential for the metabolism of lactose. The mRNA transcribed by the *lac* operon is extremely unstable, having a half-life of approximately 3 min, which means that expression of the operon can change rapidly. As soon as inducer concentrations fall, expression of the gene ceases.

The *lac* repressor

The *i* gene codes for a repressor regulatory protein, called the ***lac* repressor**, and the *i* gene itself is not regulated but continues to produce the repressor at a low level, independent of other cellular events. The *lac* repressor is expressed as a monomer of 360 amino acids, which are associated to form a tetramer, and there are usually about 10 tetramers in the cell at any one time. The tetramer binds with high affinity to a specific DNA sequence situated between the promoter called *lacP*, and the operator, called *lacO*, for the *z* gene. This binding reaction blocks the binding of RNA polymerase to the promoter. The operon is said to be **repressed**.

Derepression of the operon

Lactose induces or derepresses the operon by binding to specific high-affinity sites on the tetramer subunits. The binding reaction causes an allosteric change in the tetramer, which drastically lowers its affinity for the DNA sequence to which it usually binds.

Lactose is not the only inducer. A number of so-called gratuitous inducers have been found, including isopropylthiogalactose, which bind to the tetramer but are not themselves metabolized by β-galactosidase, and are therefore useful in the study of the *lac* operon. The mechanism described above is an example of **negative control**. But, lactose metabolism can also be under **positive control**.

POSITIVE CONTROL

E. coli prefers glucose to lactose as an energy substrate; if there is plenty of glucose in the cell, the *lac* operon is repressed, even if there is plenty of lactose present. This is known as **catabolite repression**, since it happens only when glucose is being metabolized.

The cell will turn to lactose as a substrate only when glucose concentrations fall. When concentrations of glucose are high, those of the second messenger cAMP are low. When glucose concentrations fall, concentrations of cAMP in the cell rise, and cAMP binds to a protein called **catabolite activator protein** (CAP), which is an allosteric protein. CAP undergoes a conformational change as a result of the binding reaction. This enables CAP to bind to the promoter just before the RNA polymerase binding site, and this in turn facilitates the binding of RNA polymerase to the promoter. CAP synthesis is regulated by a gene that is not a component of the *lac* operon.

CAP is an activator of a number of other genes, including the galactose and arabinose operons, and is probably a co-ordinator for the general control of enzyme synthesis whose activity is unwanted when high concentrations of the preferred energy substrate (glucose) are high.

21 Control of gene expression in eukaryotes

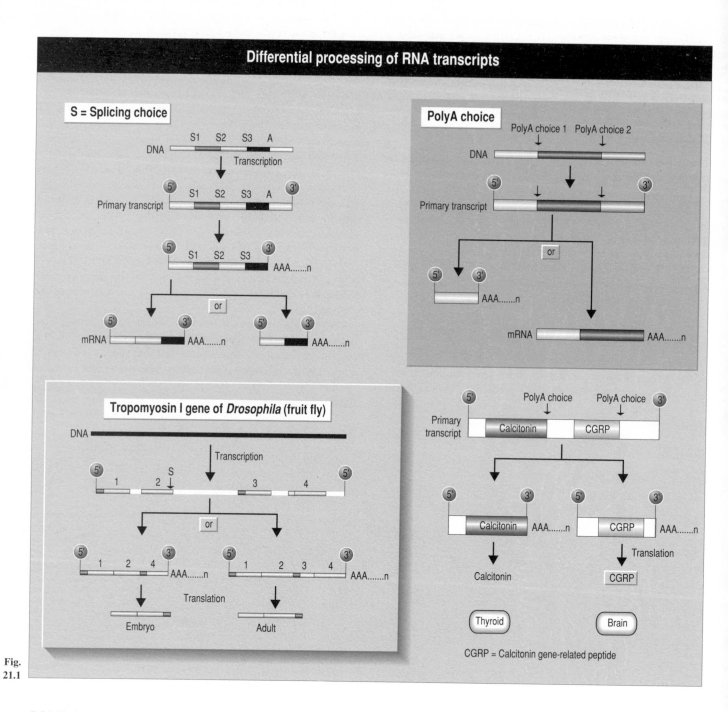

Fig. 21.1

COMPONENTS OF GENE CONTROL

Gene control has three main components: (i) signals; (ii) levels; and (iii) mechanisms. Signals include hormones, protein factors and environmental conditions such as heat shock.

Levels of regulation

Control is effected at three levels: (i) nuclear RNA synthesis; (ii) differential processing of primary transcripts; and (iii) altering mRNA stability in the cytoplasm. Control of nuclear RNA synthesis is effected mainly at the **initiation** stage. Initiation is activated by **transcription factors (activators)**, which may interact with genomic **promoters**, in order to guide RNA polymerase II to the correct site for expression of an mRNA species.

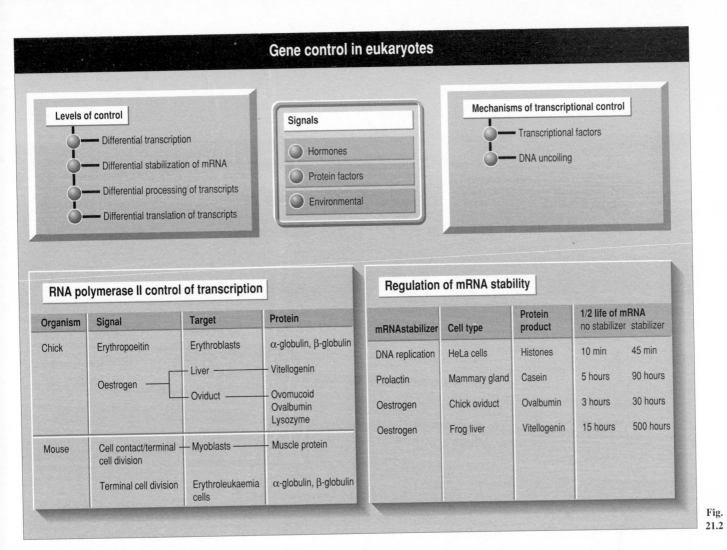

Fig. 21.2

Nuclear RNA synthesis

Cell or organism	Transcription factor	Genomic target	Cell or organism	Transcription factor	Genomic target
Mammalian cells	Sp1	Promoters containing GC boxes, e.g. dihydrofolate reductase promoter	Glucocorticoid-responsive cells	Glucocorticoid receptor	5'-GGTACA*nnn*TGTTCT-3' consensus sequence (*n*, any nucleotide); genes coding for, e.g. chicken lysozome
	CTF	CAAT box			
Drosophila	B protein	TATA box	Yeast	gal4 protein	Specific upstream sequences in promoters of genes expressing galactose-metabolizing enzymes
	HSTF	Promoter of heat shock genes			
B lymphocytes	Immunoglobulin enhancer	Enhancer sequence for immunoglobulin gene expression			

CTF, CCAAT-binding transcription factor; HSTF, heat shock transcription factor.

Differential nuclear processing of transcripts. Differential choice of **polyA sites** on the primary transcripts determines tissue specificity of gene expression. For example, in rats, the transcript encoding the hormone **calcitonin** also codes for a brain peptide, calcitonin gene-related peptide (**CGRP**), and in the thyroid gland the cells involved produce calcitonin, while in the brain CGRP is produced.

Cytoplasmic gene control. The rate of protein synthesis may be affected by: (i) the rate of transport of mRNA into the cytoplasm; (ii) half-life of mRNA; (iii) frequency of mRNA translation; and (iv) post-translational control. Control of **half-life of mRNA** may be enhanced by hormone, the occurrence of DNA replication, tissue regeneration (liver) and by certain viral proteins.

22 Mechanisms of transcriptional control

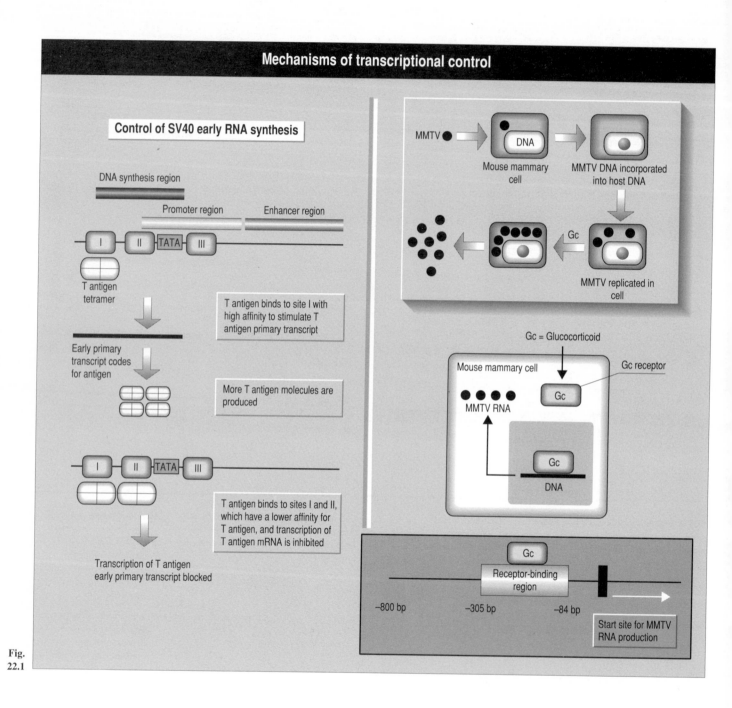

Mechanisms of transcriptional control

Control of SV40 early RNA synthesis

DNA synthesis region

Promoter region | Enhancer region

I | II | TATA | III

T antigen tetramer

T antigen binds to site I with high affinity to stimulate T antigen primary transcript

Early primary transcript codes for antigen

More T antigen molecules are produced

I | II | TATA | III

T antigen binds to sites I and II, which have a lower affinity for T antigen, and transcription of T antigen mRNA is inhibited

Transcription of T antigen early primary transcript blocked

MMTV

Mouse mammary cell

MMTV DNA incorporated into host DNA

Gc

MMTV replicated in cell

Gc = Glucocorticoid

Mouse mammary cell

MMTV RNA

Gc

Gc receptor

Gc

DNA

Gc

Receptor-binding region

−800 bp | −305 bp | −84 bp

Start site for MMTV RNA production

Fig. 22.1

INTRODUCTION

This is a brief, but more detailed look at some of the mechanisms underlying the processes whereby transcription is controlled. Examples used are the following.

1 The role of the T antigen in the control of transcription in the SV40 virus, which is a papovavirus. These are a family of small, non-enveloped double-stranded DNA viruses, including the papilloma viruses which produce the common wart, some of which can be oncogenic.

2 The role of glucocorticoids in the control of transcription of the MMTV.

SV40 VIRUS

When SV40 virus infects cells, its DNA is transcribed by host RNA polymerase II. SV40 DNA contains two transcription units: one termed 'early', and the other termed 'late'. This is because the early unit is preferentially transcribed soon after infection, and the late unit is preferentially transcribed later during infection. The shift from early to late stages is mediated by a protein called T antigen, which is produced during early transcription. T antigen, which functions as a tetramer, has three binding sites on SV40 DNA: I, II and III. Binding to I may increase the affinity of T antigen for sites II and III, thus inhibiting further transcription of the early primary transcript. T antigen may therefore be an autoregulatory protein, which inhibits the synthesis of its own mRNA. T antigen was the first of the proteins to be discovered in eukaryotes that binds to specific sites on the DNA.

MMTV

Steroids are lipophilic substances which pass easily through the plasma membrane and combine with specific receptor proteins. These complexes bind to specific sites on the DNA to alter transcription. For example, glucocorticoids are substances that bind to intracellular receptors. Glucocorticoids are known to stimulate the production of increased numbers of MMTV molecules in cells infected with the retrovirus.

> *Note*: retroviruses are enveloped, single-stranded RNA viruses, including human immunodeficiency virus (HIV), which infect cells, are converted into DNA by the enzyme reverse transcriptase. The DNA is incorporated into a host chromosome and may preferentially be transcribed back into the virus or remain dormant for several cell generations.

23 Growth

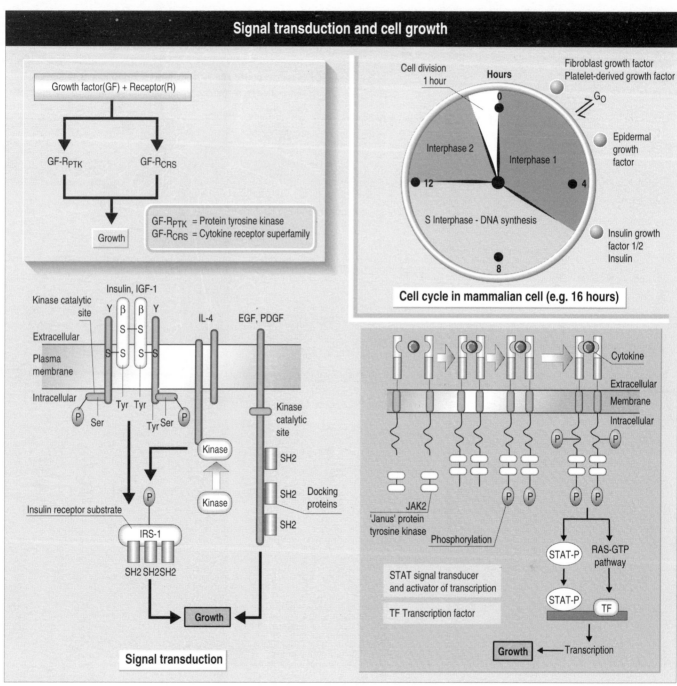

Signal transduction and cell growth

Growth factor(GF) + Receptor(R)

GF-R$_{PTK}$ GF-R$_{CRS}$

Growth

GF-R$_{PTK}$ = Protein tyrosine kinase
GF-R$_{CRS}$ = Cytokine receptor superfamily

Cell division 1 hour
Hours
Fibroblast growth factor
Platelet-derived growth factor
G$_O$
Interphase 2
Interphase 1
Epidermal growth factor
12
4
S Interphase - DNA synthesis
Insulin growth factor 1/2
Insulin
8

Cell cycle in mammalian cell (e.g. 16 hours)

Insulin, IGF-1
Kinase catalytic site
Y   β   β   Y
S—S   S—S
IL-4   EGF, PDGF
Extracellular
Plasma membrane
S—S   S—S
Intracellular
P   Tyr Tyr Tyr Ser P
Ser
Kinase catalytic site
Kinase
SH2
Kinase
SH2   Docking proteins
P
Insulin receptor substrate
IRS-1
SH2
SH2 SH2SH2
Growth

Signal transduction

Cytokine
Extracellular
Membrane
Intracellular
P   P
JAK2
'Janus' protein tyrosine kinase
Phosphorylation
P   P   P   P
STAT-P   RAS-GTP pathway
STAT signal transducer and activator of transcription
STAT-P   TF
TF Transcription factor
Growth ← Transcription

Fig. 23.1

THE CELL CYCLE

The eukaryotic cell has a life cycle characterized by four distinct successive phases, called G_1, S, G_2 and M. G stands for gap, S for synthesis and M for mitosis. DNA is synthesized during the S phase, while RNA and protein are synthesized during G_1, S and G_2. The S, G_2

and the M phases in different growing cells remain relatively constant in duration (7, 3 and 1 h, respectively). During mitosis, RNA synthesis ceases and protein synthesis is greatly reduced.

Mitosis is a typical process of nuclear division, when two daughter nuclei are formed, each having the same chromosomal complement as the parent nucleus. **Cell** division occurs after a full cycle has been

Growth factor or hormone*	Main sources	Target tissue or cell
EGF	Mouse submaxillary gland	Epidermal cells, fibroblasts
Transforming growth factor α (TGF-α)	Embryonic and cancerous cells	e.g. fibroblasts
TGF–β	Most cells, cancer cells	e.g. fibroblasts
Erythropoeitin	Kidney	Red blood cell precursors (erythroblasts)
Insulin	Pancreatic islet	Liver, muscle
Nerve growth factor (NGF)	Many cells	Sympathetic nerves
PDGF	Platelets	Arterial smooth muscle cells (repair function)
IGF–II; somatomedin A	Liver	Mediates GH action on growing bone; mitogenic in some cells
GH	Anterior pituitary	Liver–stimulates somatomedin production

*This list is not comprehensive.

completed. Some cells, such as muscle and nerve, may never divide after formation, while others, such as liver, skin or gut, will be active in cell division. When the cell enters a phase called G_0, it is dormant until a trigger (usually a growth factor) switches it into active cell division. Certain growth factors, notably platelet–derived growth factor (PDGF), fibroblast growth factor (FGF), epidermal growth factor (EGF), and insulin-like growth factor (IGF–1) and IGF–2 (see below), stimulate the cell cycle at various points during G_1.

GROWTH FACTORS

Growth factors are peptides that stimulate cellular proliferation. They regulate normal growth and development. They may also cause what is known as phenotypic transformation of cells, which may result in cancer. They produce these effects through an interaction with a specific receptor on the cell surface. They fall into several arbitrarily classified groups.

1 **Hormones**, such as **insulin,** secreted by the B cells of the pancreas, **growth hormone** (GH) and **prolactin**, both of which are secreted by the anterior pituitary gland.

2 **Cytokines**, which are not necessarily hormones, and which are made by many different cells. They affect growth and division of cells.

3 **Lymphokines**, which are polypeptides released by activated macrophages and T cells of the immune system. Some influence white cell migration, while others also act as growth factors. Interleukin 1 (IL-1), which is released by macrophages, stimulates proliferation and differentiation of the B lymphocytes.

Mechanicsm of action of growth factors

Growth factors exert their effects on cells through **membrane receptors**. When the factor binds to the receptor, the signal is transferred to the cell in the form of a cascade of several reactions, especially phosphorylation reactions. In certain cases, the intracellular domain of the receptor contains a protein kinase that enables the receptor to autophosphorylate itself (see below). The final result is initiation of transcription, protein synthesis and growth.

The growth factor receptors can be classified in terms of the intracellular phosphorylation cascade.

Insulin receptor substrate 1 (IRS-1) signalling system. Some hormones and growth factors, for example insulin and IGF-I, bind to receptors that contain intrinsic tyrosine kinase activity and autophosphorylate themselves. This results in the tyrosine phosphorylation of a protein called IRS-1. This enables a group of so-called SH2 proteins (proteins with *src* homology) to 'dock' at IRS-1, resulting in consequent

intracellular events culminating in the mitogenic response. Some growth factors, e.g. **IL-4**, bind to a receptor that does not contain intrinsic kinase activity, but which recruits a cytoplasmic tyrosine kinase that phosphorylates IRS-1 on tyrosine to create the SH2 binding sites.

Note: the insulin receptor consists of two α-chains, each of which binds a molecule of insulin, and two β-chains., which span the membrane and contain the catalytic sites. The chains are held together by disulphide bonds.

Receptor kinase–SH2 system. Certain growth factors, for example EGF and PDGF, bind to receptors that possess intrinsic kinase activity, which allows them to become autophosphorylated, and these phosphorylated sites become docking sites for SH2 proteins.

Cytokine receptor superfamily (CRS). This is a group of hormone and growth factor receptors that do not themselves have any kinase activity, but which activate a group of cytoplasmic protein kinase kinases, called the **Janus kinase (JAK)** family. At least four members of the JAK family have been identified: JAK1, JAK2, JAK3 and TYK2, and there are probably more. The JAK proteins bind to the membrane proximal area of the activated receptor, become tyrosine phosphorylated and in turn they phosphorylate the receptor causing the activation of the following.

1 A group of cytoplasmic proteins that form part of a family of transcription activators, called **signal transducers and transcription activators (STATS).**

2 The phosphorylated STATS activate transcription at the level of the DNA — the **Ras** pathway. The phosphorylated receptor provides binding sites for a group of SH2 docking proteins, which activates the Ras–GTP system, resulting in activation of a group of mitogen-activated protein kinase (MAPK), and a transcription activator TF.

Termination of action

Growth factor action will be terminated by the dissociation of the factor from its binding site on the receptor. It may also be terminated by the inactivation of the intracellular MAPK. There is evidence that the MAPK may be down-regulated by dephosphorylating enzyme phosphatases. Furthermore, it seems that when MAPK are activated this triggers the expression of the genes encoding the phosphatases, which would provide a tightly and elegantly controlled mechanism for the regulation of growth factor activity. Any disturbance of this control system might conceivably contribute to the factors that cause cancer through unrestrained growth factor action.

24 Cancer

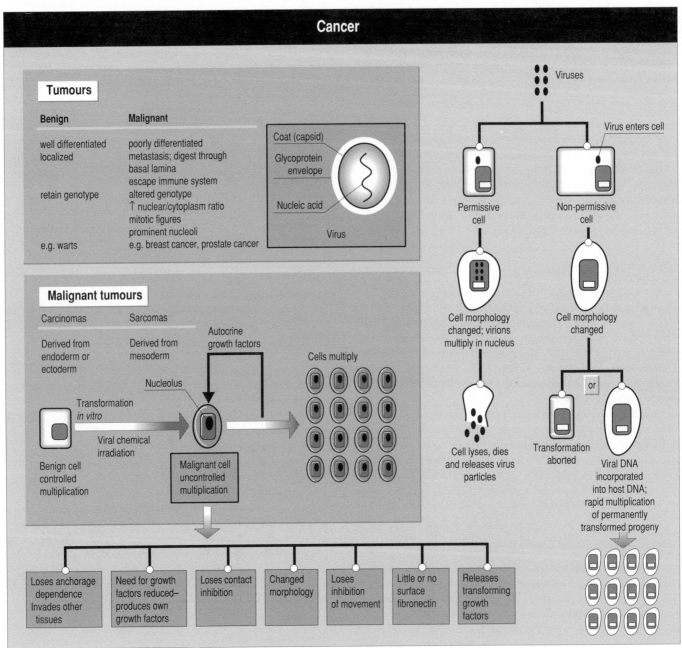

Fig. 24.1

Cancer is the uncontrolled, apparently autonomous growth of cells, and their invasion of the rest of the body. Such cells are termed **malignant**, and their invasion is termed **metastasis**. Normal cells become transformed through **mutagenic** agents.

MALIGNANCY

Knowledge of the molecular basis of cancer stems largely from the study of **viral** activation of **oncogenes**.

Cancer-producing viruses

Certain viruses transform healthy cells to malignancy. Viruses are

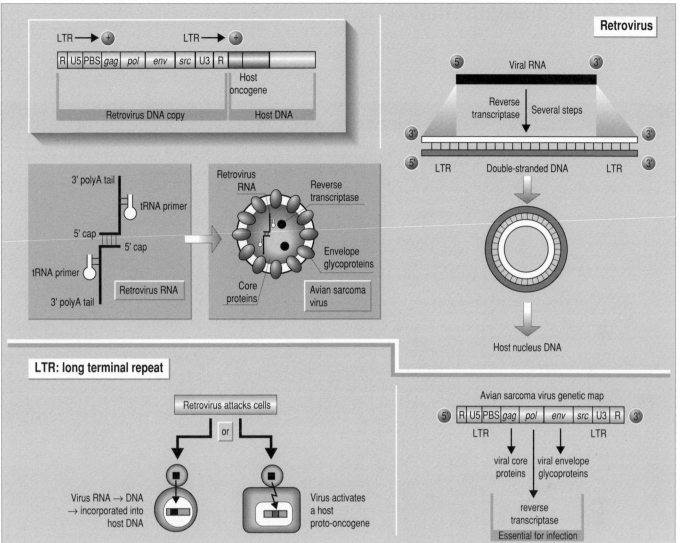

Fig.
24.2

infectious DNA or RNA, which may be single or double stranded, surrounded by a protective coat consisting of a large number of repeating protein subunits.

Viruses must invade other cells to multiply, and their own nucleic acid instructs the host (permissive) cell to synthesize more viral nucleic acid protein. This invasion usually kills the cell, and the complete **virion**, or virus particle, is released. Occasionally, the cell is non-permissive, and may destroy the invading virus, or incorporate the viral genetic information into its own genome.

Some viruses that contain RNA are termed **retroviruses**. They have a polymerase enzyme termed **reverse transcriptase**, which, when they have entered a cell, produces a double-stranded DNA copy which is incorporated into host DNA. The cell is transformed either because the viral DNA copy contains the oncogene, or because the viral genes activate a host oncogene.

The avian sarcoma retrovirus binds to specific cell membrane receptors, and inserts its contents into the cell. Reverse transcriptase produces a DNA copy which is longer than the viral RNA template because it contains **long terminal repeats** (**LTR**). The LTR contains the enhancers, polyadenylation sites and promoters. The viral DNA circularizes, enters the host nucleus, and is spliced into the host DNA at TCAG sites.

The 10 kbp of avian sarcoma virus contains four genes, three of which are necessary for infection. These are *gag*, *pol* and *env*. The other, *src*, is necessary for transformation to occur. Three viral mRNA species are expressed: one unspliced mRNA coding for both *gag* and *pol*; and two unspliced mRNAs encoding *env* and *src*. The *src* product is a tyrosine kinase. The viral proteins and the unspliced primary RNA transcript migrate to the cell membrane and are incorporated into it. Part of the altered membrane buds off a new viral particle. Retroviruses do not usually kill the host. The HIV is a retrovirus.

Oncogenes

Oncogenes are cancer-producing genes. They may be present on the viral genome, imported into the host genome or already present as a cellular gene which is activated through viral infection. Cellular oncogenes (also called **proto-oncogenes**) are usually silent, or expressed normally under cellular control. But, if a viral DNA copy is spliced into the cellular genome adjacent to a proto-oncogene, the viral LTR may stimulate its expression, thereby transforming the cell.

Oncogenes are named after the species and disease produced by the infective virus.

25 Genetic manipulation I

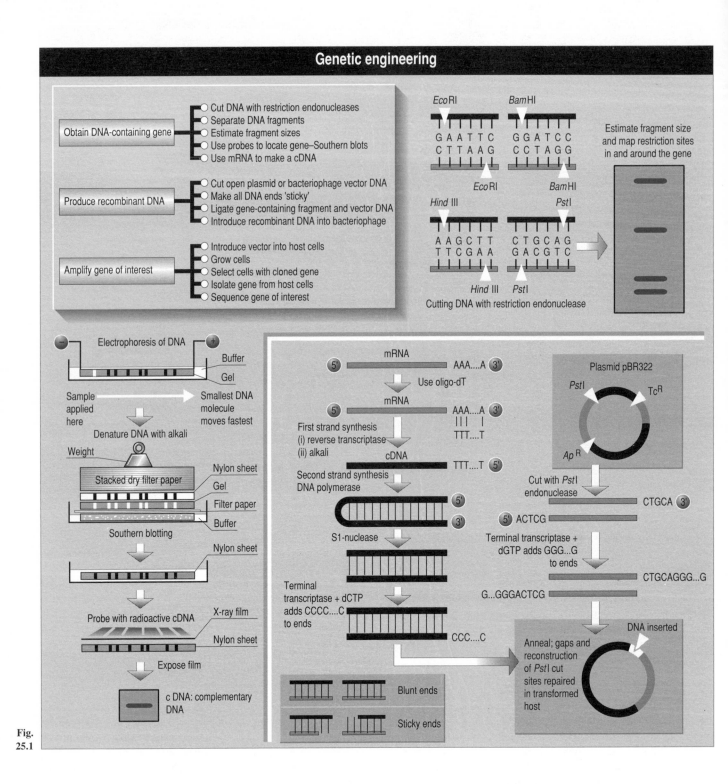

Genetic engineering

Obtain DNA-containing gene
- Cut DNA with restriction endonucleases
- Separate DNA fragments
- Estimate fragment sizes
- Use probes to locate gene–Southern blots
- Use mRNA to make a cDNA

Produce recombinant DNA
- Cut open plasmid or bacteriophage vector DNA
- Make all DNA ends 'sticky'
- Ligate gene-containing fragment and vector DNA
- Introduce recombinant DNA into bacteriophage

Amplify gene of interest
- Introduce vector into host cells
- Grow cells
- Select cells with cloned gene
- Isolate gene from host cells
- Sequence gene of interest

*Eco*RI
G A A T T C
C T T A A G
*Eco*RI

*Bam*HI
G G A T C C
C C T A G G
*Bam*HI

Hind III
A A G C T T
T T C G A A
Hind III

*Pst*I
C T G C A G
G A C G T C
*Pst*I

Cutting DNA with restriction endonuclease

Estimate fragment size and map restriction sites in and around the gene

Electrophoresis of DNA
Buffer
Gel
Sample applied here
Smallest DNA molecule moves fastest

Denature DNA with alkali
Weight
Nylon sheet
Stacked dry filter paper
Gel
Filter paper
Buffer

Southern blotting
Nylon sheet

Probe with radioactive cDNA
X-ray film
Nylon sheet

Expose film

c DNA: complementary DNA

mRNA
5' ————— AAA....A 3'
Use oligo-dT

mRNA
5' ————— AAA....A 3'
||| |
TTT....T

First strand synthesis
(i) reverse transcriptase
(ii) alkali

cDNA
TTT....T 5'

Second strand synthesis
DNA polymerase
5'
3'

S1-nuclease

Terminal transcriptase + dCTP adds CCCC....C to ends
CCC....C

Blunt ends
Sticky ends

Plasmid pBR322
*Pst*I
Tc^R
Ap^R

Cut with *Pst*I endonuclease
CTGCA 3'
5' ACTCG

Terminal transcriptase + dGTP adds GGG...G to ends
CTGCAGGG...G
G...GGGACTCG

Anneal; gaps and reconstruction of *Pst*I cut sites repaired in transformed host
DNA inserted

Fig. 25.1

INTRODUCTION

Genetic manipulation is the alteration of DNA, which is transmitted in a vector system into host organisms, in which the manipulated gene(s) are amplified and recovered for further use. The genes implanted into the host may cause it to express the gene products directed by the implanted gene. The vector may be a bacterial plasmid, a bacteriophage, or the DNA may be introduced directly into mammalian embryonic tissues using surgical techniques.

Techniques involve the introduction of the chosen DNA nucleotide sequence into a vector, the introduction of the vector into a host in which the sequence will be amplified, the cloning of the altered host and the recovery of the amplified sequence.

CREATING THE DNA SEQUENCE

DNA from mRNA

The production of a mixture of **cDNA** from small quantities of mRNA is made possible using the enzyme **reverse transcriptase**, obtained from retroviruses. Double-stranded DNA for insertion into a vector can be prepared from the mRNA expressed by the gene. The **procedure** involves the following.

1 The mRNA is isolated and given an oligo (d)T primer, after which it is incubated with reverse transcriptase and the four deoxynucleotides to make the first cDNA strand.

2 The first strand has at its 3′ end a hairpin bend which is used, together with a primer called the **Klenow fragment** and DNA polymerase to make a second DNA strand complementary to the first, after which the bend is removed with an enzyme, S1 nuclease.

3 The 3′-terminal ends of the DNA are given homopolymeric tracts of CCC..., etc., which combine non-covalently with tracts of GGG..., etc., added to ends of a cut plasmid. After the plasmid with its new addition of the sequence of interest is annealed, it is introduced into the host.

It is possible to amplify the gene starting with minutely small quantities of mRNA. A disadvantage is that many thousands of different cDNA molecules will be cloned.

Restriction endonucleases

Cutting DNA at selected sites is possible through the use of restriction endonucleases. The physiological role of these enzymes is to destroy unwanted cellular DNA. Once DNA has been extracted, it can be cut with enzymes that recognize certain sequences, and which cut the tracts in predictable places. The enzymes share in common the ability to read palindromic sequences. (A pure **palindrome**, e.g. AATTAA, is identical when read from left to right or from right to left.) Some enzymes (e.g. AluI) cut the DNA leaving 'blunt' ends. This is not ideal, since a meeting between ends to be joined depends purely on chance. Some enzymes (e.g. EcoRI) make 'sticky' ends, with sequences extending from the chain, allowing complementary base pairing with another chain.

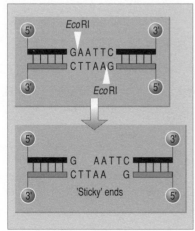

Fig.
25.2

SEPARATION OF DNA FRAGMENTS

Restriction endonucleases will cut the DNA into several fragments of differing sizes. These are separated by gel electrophoresis. The negatively charged DNA fragments migrate to the positive electrodes, with the smallest moving fastest. In order to estimate the sizes, a separate lane is run containing standard DNA fragments of known size. After electrophoresis, the bands of separated DNA are visualized by staining the gel with ethidium bromide, which intercalates in the DNA and fluoresces under UV light. The gel can be photographed. This enables the estimation of the number of fragments cut. As little as 25 ng of DNA can be seen this way. If the starting DNA material is radioactively labelled with phosphorus-32 (^{32}P), 1–2 ng of DNA can be visualized using X-ray film. The size of the band is obtained by comparison with the migration rate of the standards.

Once the size and number of fragments are known, and the sites where they have been cut, it is possible to start constructing a map of the DNA molecule — so-called gene maps.

SOUTHERN BLOTTING AND GENE PROBING

The technique of blotting involves transferring the separated DNA bands from the gel to a nitrocellulose or nylon sheet, when the DNA bands are transferred by capillary action. Once on the sheet, the DNA is fixed to it by heating or chemical reaction, and the bands can be probed using a radioactively labelled gene probe, whose DNA sequence is complementary to that of the gene to be probed for. The probe hybridizes to the gene, the unbound probe is washed away and the hybridized probe visualized. The experiment confirms that a gene has indeed been isolated. The DNA of interest can be recovered and inserted into a vector.

RNA can be electrophoresed instead of DNA, and transferred to a nitrocellulose or nylon sheet (**Northern blotting**); the separated bands of RNA are probed with labelled cDNA complementary to the mRNA expressed. This confirms that a particular gene has been expressed, and that its mRNA is among the species of mRNA electrophoresed. Similarly, proteins can be transferred and probed using immunocyto-chemical techniques, when the process is termed **Western blotting**.

POLYMERASE CHAIN REACTION (PCR)

PCR enables us to amplify very rapidly a DNA sequence in a small biological sample. This allows the identification of potential disease-producing genes in a prenatal sample, the forensic identification of DNA for legal purposes and the amplification of sequences for insertion into vectors or for sequencing purposes.

Principle

The method was made possible by the discovery of organisms living near boiling geysers. Their enzymes, including DNA polymerase, operate at high temperatures. PCR depends on the use of this DNA polymerase, a supply of the four (d) nucleotides and primers which flank the DNA to be amplified, after it has been denatured to give single-stranded DNA: (i) the DNA is denatured at 90°C; (ii) the primers anneal to the sequence to be amplified at 50°C; (iii) the primer sequences are extended at 70°C; (iv) the cycle is repeated several times; and (v) the amplified DNA is recovered from the reaction mix. Theoretically, it is possible to create over 250 million copies after 30 cycles.

26 **Genetic manipulation II**

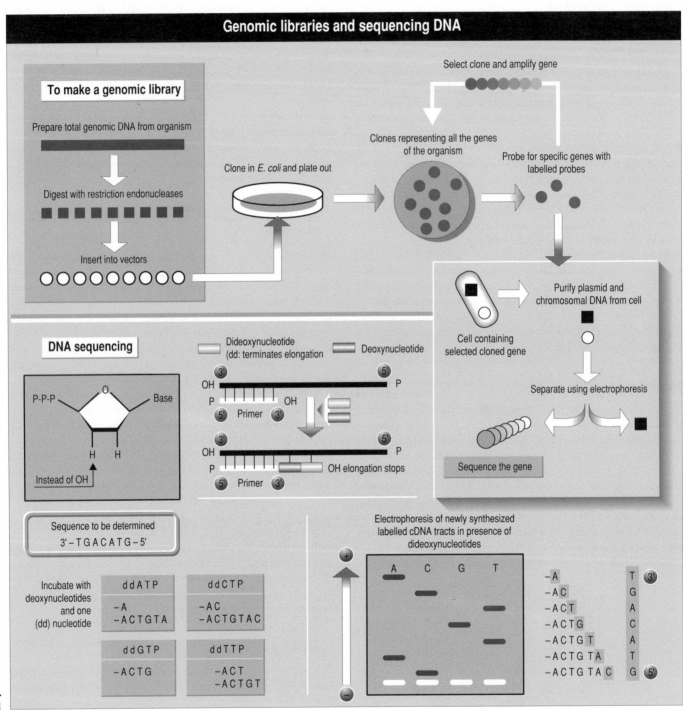

Genomic libraries and sequencing DNA

To make a genomic library

Prepare total genomic DNA from organism

Digest with restriction endonucleases

Insert into vectors

Clone in *E. coli* and plate out

Clones representing all the genes of the organism

Select clone and amplify gene

Probe for specific genes with labelled probes

Cell containing selected cloned gene

Purify plasmid and chromosomal DNA from cell

Separate using electrophoresis

Sequence the gene

DNA sequencing

P-P-P   O   Base

H   H

Instead of OH

Dideoxynucleotide (dd: terminates elongation)   Deoxynucleotide

OH   P

Primer

OH   P

OH elongation stops

Primer

Sequence to be determined
3' – T G A C A T G – 5'

Incubate with deoxynucleotides and one (dd) nucleotide

ddATP	ddCTP
–A –ACTGTA	–AC –ACTGTAC

ddGTP	ddTTP
–ACTG	–ACT –ACTGT

Electrophoresis of newly synthesized labelled cDNA tracts in presence of dideoxynucleotides

A   C   G   T

–A	T 3'
–AC	G
–ACT	A
–ACTG	C
–ACTGT	A
–ACTGTA	T
–ACTGTAC	G 5'

Fig. 26.1

VECTORS

A vector must be able to enter a cell, be stable and able to replicate within the cell. The ideal vector has a low molecular weight, enters host cells easily, readily confers selected phenotype characteristics on host cells and possesses single sites for many restriction endonucleases.

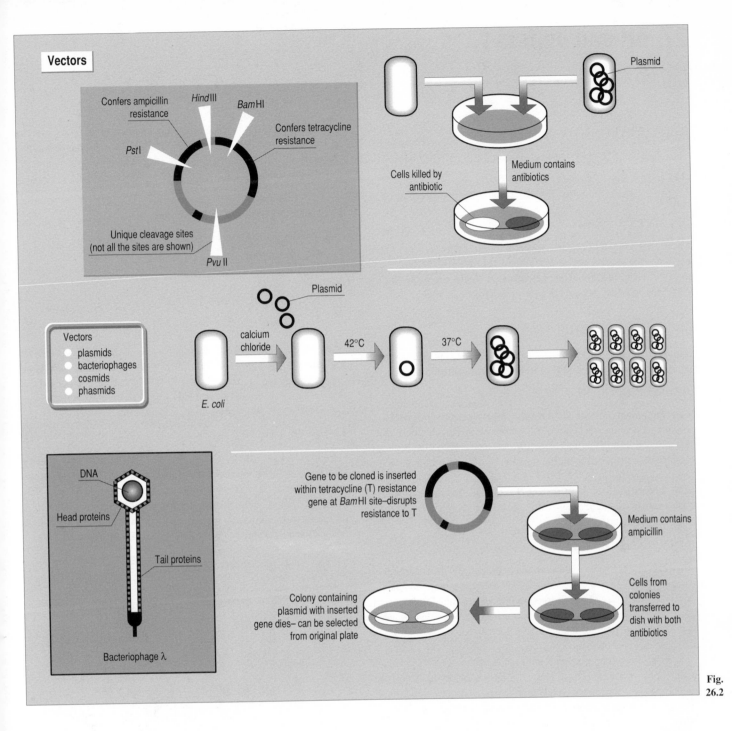

Fig. 26.2

Plasmids

Plasmids are small circular DNA, occurring naturally in bacteria. Inside bacteria, plasmids replicate independently of the chromosomal DNA. Plasmids enter bacterial cells more readily if the cells are first treated with $CaCl_2$ at low temperatures, or exposed to an electric field ('electroporation'). $CaCl_2$ causes the plasmid to bind to the cell membrane, and if the cell is heated briefly to 40°C, the plasmid rapidly enters the cell. Transformed cells, i.e. those containing foreign DNA, will replicate in culture to form a **clone** of daughter cells. Not all the bacteria in a culture will take up the plasmid that contains the gene of interest; these have to be distinguished and separated from those that have taken up the gene. Plasmids, such as pBR322, have been designed to achieve this separation.

pBR322. Plasmid pBR322 is an artificial circular DNA molecule containing 4363 base pairs, and contains sequences which are the genes which confer resistance to ampicillin and tetracycline (genes Ap^R and Tc^R, respectively). The plasmid also has several sites for cleavage by restriction endonucleases. When the plasmid is cleaved, the size of every fragment produced can be calculated.

Other vectors

Bacteriophages are viruses that infect bacteria. The phage binds to the bacterial membrane and injects its nucleic acid into the cell, where it is replicated. The phage can be 'primed' with the recombinant DNA one wants to infect the cell with.

27 pH and buffers I

DISSOCIATION OF H_2O

The dissociation of H_2O is through a breakage of an –OH bond:

$$H_2O \rightleftharpoons H^+ + OH^- \tag{1}$$

at 25°C:

$$[H^+][OH^-] = 10^{-14} \text{ mol/l}^2 \tag{2}$$

where $[H^+]$ and $[OH^-]$ are the concentrations of the two ions in moles per litre. The relative molecular mass of H_2O is 18; therefore, 1 mol of H_2O weighs 18 g. One litre of H_2O weighs 1000 g. Therefore, H_2O is $1000/18 \approx 56$ mol/l. In pure H_2O, $[H^+] = [OH^-] = 10^{-7}$ mol/l.

pH

It is more convenient to refer to the hydrogen ion concentration in whole numbers. To do this, –log of $[H^+]$ is used (–log is called 'p'). Thus:

$$pH = -\log[H^+] \tag{3}$$

Therefore, when $[H^+] = [OH^-]$, the pH = 7, i.e. the neutral pH. Below 7, solutions are acidic, and above 7, solutions are basic (alkaline). Note that a change of 1 pH unit means a 10-fold change in $[H^+]$. In the body the pH varies, depending on the function of the compartment. In the cell cytoplasm the pH is 7.2. In the stomach, where food is digested by acid, the pH is about 1. In the small intestine it is about 8, and in lysosomes it is about 5.

ACIDS AND BASES

An acid is any molecule that can release a proton, and gains a negative charge, and a base is a substance that can accept a proton, and gain a positive charge. Negatively charged molecules are called **anions**, and positively charged molecules are called **cations**. **Strong acids** are acids that readily lose protons and are 100% dissociated, and **strong bases** are those that take them up.

In an acidic solution, a **weak acid** (such as the –COOH group of amino acids or the phosphate groups of nucleic acids) tends to hold onto its protons (i.e. remain largely unionized), while a **weak base** will take up protons (i.e. ionize). In a basic solution, weak acids will ionize, while weak bases are only partially ionized.

Nucleic acids ionize by releasing protons, and become negatively charged. Amino acids contain both basic (–NH$_2$) and acidic (–COOH) groups, and can become positively or negatively charged, or both.

Ionization of amino acids

Amino acids have –COOH groups which can release protons, and they have –NH$_2$ groups which can accept protons. Therefore, depending on the pH of the solution, amino acids can exist as weak acids or bases. Since proteins may have unequally balanced numbers of –COOH and –NH$_2$ groups, changes in pH of the solution in which they are dissolved will cause changes in the ratio of charged acidic and basic groups. For different amino acids, the pH at which the –COOH and

–NH$_2$ groups exactly balance each other to create no net charge on the molecule is called the isoelectric pH of the molecule. In chemical terms, any molecule that has both negatively and positively charged groups is called a **zwitterion**.

The Henderson–Hasselbalch equation

The –COOH group ionizes thus:

$$COOH \rightleftharpoons COO^- + H^+ \tag{5}$$

At equilibrium:

$$K = \frac{[COO^-][H^+]}{[COOH]} \tag{6}$$

where **K** (also sometimes called Ka) is the equilibrium constant for Equation (5). **pK** is defined as the pH at which 50% of the –COOH (or –NH$_2$) groups are ionized. Clearly, K will depend on the numbers of these groups that the amino acid has.

Similarly, the –NH$_3^+$ group is deprotonated thus:

$$NH_3^+ \rightleftharpoons NH_2 + H^+ \tag{7}$$

Figure 27.1 is a titration curve for the –COOH and –NH$_2$ groups, showing that deprotonation of the groups occurs over a pH range, and the pH at which 50% of the groups are deprotonated is the pK. Note that at pH values below the pK, the protonated form predominates; at pH values above the pK, the deprotonated forms predominate. It follows that a stronger acid has a lower pK, i.e. it readily loses protons.

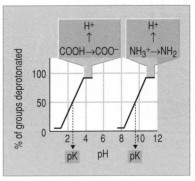

Fig. 27.1

Using Equation (6), we can derive one which enables us to predict the state of ionization of a given amino acid if we know K and the pH of the solution.

1 Rearrange and take the log of both sides

$$\log K = \log[H^+] + \log \frac{[COO^-]}{[COOH]} \tag{8}$$

2 Convert to –log and rearrange

$$-\log[H^+] = -\log[K] + \log \frac{[COO^-]}{[COOH]} \tag{9}$$

3 Express in terms of p(–log): the **Henderson–Hasselbalch equation**

$$pH = pK + \log\frac{[COO^-]}{[COOH]} \qquad (10)$$

Equation (10) allows us to predict, for example, the degree of ionization of the –COOH group of drugs for absorption through biological membranes, which are lipophilic and allow only the unionized form of the drug to pass through easily. For example, aspirin is a weak acid, with a pK of 3.5; the reader is invited to use Equation (10) to calculate the degree of ionization, i.e. the ratio of ionized to unionized groups in the stomach (pH 1.5), and in the small intestine (pH 8). From this result, the theoretical site of greater absorption may be predicted.

BUFFERS

Buffer solutions are those that resist a change in pH even when H^+ ions are added to, or removed from the solution. Thus, they protect the solutes within the buffer from sharp changes in pH that could, for example, inhibit a chemical reaction. In the absence of a buffering mechanism, the pH of a solution will change much more when acids or alkalis are added to the solution.

Mechanism of buffer action

The weak acid, acetic acid (CH_3COOH) (found in vinegar and bad wine), and its salt sodium acetate (CH_3COONa) provide an example of a buffering system. The acid has a pK of 4.75. A change of 2 pH units in the solution from 5.75 to 3.75 causes a change from about 10% CH_3COOH in the unionized form to about 90% unionized CH_3COOH. The ability of a weak acid and its salt to buffer a solution is greatest over the pH range pK –1 to pK +1. When CH_3COOH and CH_3COONa are present together in solution, they ionize as follows:

$$CH_3COOH \rightleftharpoons CH_3COO^- + H^+ \qquad (11)$$

$$CH_3COONa \rightleftharpoons CH_3COO^- + Na^+ \qquad (12)$$

Although the acid ionizes only partially, salts ionize virtually completely. Therefore, there will be a large concentration of CH_3COO^- and Na^+ ions in solution. The increased concentration of CH_3COO^- ions from the salt suppresses even further the ionization of CH_3COOH. If more H^+ ions are added to the solution, they will combine with CH_3COO^- ions to form even more of the largely undissociated CH_3COOH. A new equilibrium is established, and the resulting liberation of H^+ ions is relatively slight.

If OH^- ions are added, they will combine with H^+ ions to form neutral H_2O. Thus, at pH values close to its pK, a weak acid is a useful buffering agent when mixed with its salt.

The system will lose its buffering capacity sharply at pH values more than 1 pH value away from the pK. In a strongly basic solution the weak acid itself ionizes virtually completely, so cannot exist in the unionized form, and in strongly acidic solutions it cannot exist in the ionized form.

In cells, buffering of physiological fluids is achieved largely through the ionization of phosphoric acid (H_3PO_4), to form phosphates. H_3PO_4 can exist in three forms, depending on the pH of the solution:

$$pK \approx 2.1 \qquad H_3PO_4 \rightleftharpoons H_2PO_4^- + H^+ \qquad (13)$$

$$pK \approx 7.2 \qquad H_2PO_4^- \rightleftharpoons HPO_4^{2-} + H^+ \qquad (14)$$

$$pK \approx 12.7 \qquad HPO_4^{2-} \rightleftharpoons PO_4^{3-} + H^+ \qquad (15)$$

At cytoplasmic pH, phosphates can act as buffering systems.

28 pH and buffers II

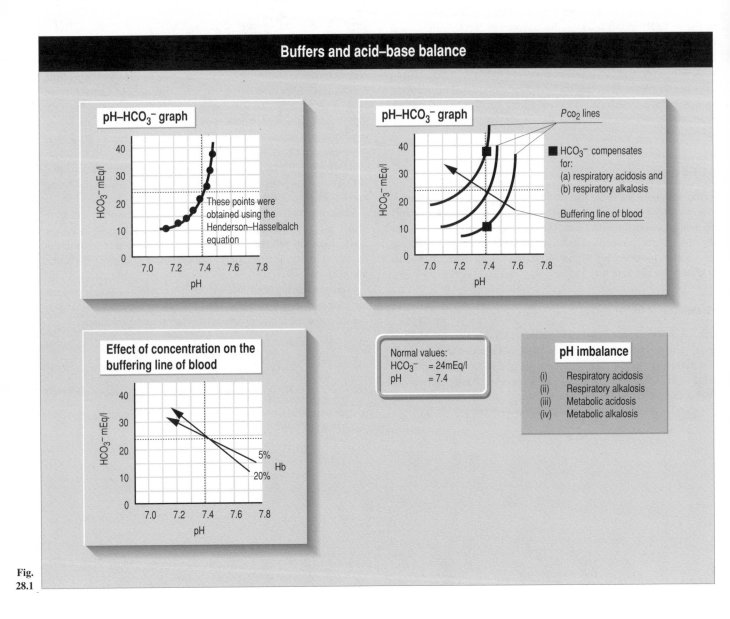

Buffers and acid–base balance

pH–HCO₃⁻ graph

These points were obtained using the Henderson–Hasselbalch equation

pH–HCO₃⁻ graph

Pco₂ lines

■ HCO₃⁻ compensates for:
(a) respiratory acidosis and
(b) respiratory alkalosis

Buffering line of blood

Effect of concentration on the buffering line of blood

5% Hb
20%

Normal values:
HCO₃⁻ = 24mEq/l
pH = 7.4

pH imbalance

(i) Respiratory acidosis
(ii) Respiratory alkalosis
(iii) Metabolic acidosis
(iv) Metabolic alkalosis

Fig. 28.1

PHYSIOLOGICAL BUFFER SYSTEMS

The major fluid compartments in the body are the intracellular fluid (ICF), and the extracellular fluid (ECF), which consists of the plasma and the interstitial fluid. All are bounded by semi-permeable membranes, whose properties depend on their function. All need buffering systems, which depend on the major ions of the compartment.

Plasma buffering system

In plasma and interstitial fluid, the CO_2–bicarbonate (HCO_3^-) system is very important. It prevents the development of dangerous acid or base imbalance, and works as follows:

$$CO_2 + H_2O \rightleftharpoons H_2CO_3 \tag{1}$$

Carbonic acid (H_2CO_3) is a weak acid, and ionizes:

$$H_2CO_3 \rightleftharpoons H^+ + HCO_3^- \tag{2}$$

H_2CO_3 ionizes so rapidly that for our purposes the reaction of importance can be considered to be:

$$CO_2 + H_2O \rightleftharpoons H^+ + HCO_3^- \tag{3}$$

Recalling the Henderson–Hasselbalch equation:

$$pH = pKa + \log \frac{[HCO_3^-]}{[CO_2][H_2O]} \tag{4}$$

The pH in blood is 7.4 (actually ranges from 7.35 to 7.45); the pKa for

HCO_3^- is 6.1. Therefore, from the previous spread, we know that this is a buffering system that operates over the pH range of about 5–7. [H_2O] is taken as unity. The concentrations of gases in fluids such as plasma are expressed as partial pressures (e.g. the P_{CO_2} in plasma ranges from 4.5 to 6.1 kPa). To convert partial pressures into concentration terms, it is necessary to use a conversion factor. For CO_2, the correction factor, at 37°C, is 0.23 mEq/l per kPa. For our purposes, let P_{CO_2} = 5.0 kPa.

From Equation (4):

$$0.4 = 6.1 + \log \frac{[HCO_3^-]}{[0.23 \times 5.0]} \qquad (5)$$

Therefore, under these conditions, [HCO_3^-] = 22.94 mEq/l.

The reader may have noticed that HCO_3^- is not, theoretically, a good buffering system above pH 7.1. Yet, it is efficient at buffering plasma at pH values as high as 7.9. This is because the body eliminates CO_2 through respiration. In other words, undissociated weak acid is being eliminated, and so Equation (3) is driven to the left. This enhances the buffering capacity of the system.

If CO_2 built up in the plasma and other tissues, the body would suffer an acidosis, but CO_2 is lost through the lungs. The pH–HCO_3^- graph shows how HCO_3^- ion changes with pH at a given P_{CO_2}. When P_{CO_2} changes, the graph shifts in a line called the **blood buffering line**. The buffering action of HCO_3^- is supplemented by proteins and phosphates, which assist to 'mop up' H^+ ions as they are formed. The steeper the slope of the buffering line, the better the buffering action. The slope reflects the concentration of Hb in blood.

Hb is an important buffering agent in blood through its transporting of CO_2, and its ionization. Hb removes about 60% of H^+ ions produced through normal CO_2 transport. Therefore, in disease states involving a depletion of Hb, the buffering capacity of the blood will be reduced.

ACID–BASE BALANCE

The body generates acids through metabolism and respiration. The major respiratory acid is CO_2, and important metabolic acids are lactic acid, and the ketoacids β-hydroxybutyric acid and acetoacetic acid. In addition, acids may be taken in the form of drugs such as aspirin (acetylsalicylic acid). In the disease state diabetes mellitus (see below) excess ketoacids are produced.

Acid–base imbalance

There are four main types of imbalance.

1 Respiratory acidosis. Here, CO_2 is retained, either because of hypoventilation or intrinsic lung disease interfering with gas exchange. For example, hypoventilation may result from depression of the respiratory centre by drugs, while intrinsic lung disease could include conditions such as chronic bronchitis. In the latter condition, mucosal thickening and airway plugging with mucus may lead to poor alveolar ventilation and CO_2 retention with low arterial P_{O_2} values.

2 Respiratory alkalosis. This results from hyperventilation. CO_2 is blown off through the lungs too rapidly, and blood pH rises. Hyperventilation may be caused by poisoning with acids such as aspirin, by fever or by anxiety.

3 Metabolic acidosis. This may arise from ingestion of acids or substances metabolized to acids (e.g. methanol intoxication, when methanol is oxidized to formic acid); from overproduction of endogenous acids such as ketoacids in diabetes mellitus; from failure to excrete non-volatile acids in certain types of renal disease, including acute and chronic renal failure; from loss of base (HCO_3^-) reserve, for example in severe diarrhoea; or from loss of alkaline upper gastrointestinal contents after surgery (e.g. fistula formation).

4 Metabolic alkalosis. This can occur through ingestion of bases such as sodium bicarbonate. It can also occur if certain diuretics are taken. Diuretics are drugs that promote the flow of urine.

The body compensates for metabolic acidosis by hyperventilation to blow off CO_2, and by increased renal (kidney) excretion of H^+ and HCO_3^- regeneration. The body compensates for metabolic alkalosis by hypoventilation and increased excretion of bicarbonate through the kidneys, although hypoventilation is limited by the fall in arterial P_{O_2} which would otherwise occur.

29 Chemical reactions I

CHEMICAL EQUILIBRIUM

A reversible chemical reaction can be characterized thus:

$$A + B \rightleftharpoons C + D \qquad (1)$$

where A and B are reactants, and C and D are products. Initially, the concentrations of C and D are low, but as their concentrations build up, so the reaction slows down, until there is no further net change in the concentrations of any of the chemicals. The reaction has reached a **chemical equilibrium** for the conditions, i.e. temperature and pressure, under which the reaction occurred, and the ratio of reactants and products is constant, defined by the **equilibrium constant** (K_{eq}):

$$K_{eq} = \left(\frac{[C]\,[D]}{[A]\,[B]} \right)_{eq} \qquad (2)$$

where [A] and [B] are the molar concentrations of reactants, and [C] and [D] are the molar concentrations of the products.

K_{eq} is useful, since it defines the reaction system under given conditions, but it does not tell whether the reaction is going to occur or not. For that, we need to know the **energy level** at the start of the reaction, and the energy level of the system at the end of the reaction.

FREE ENERGY

Free energy is the energy available for a reaction, and the relative free energies in a system at the start and end of a reaction will determine whether a reaction will take place or not. In other words, it is the **change in free energy** (ΔG) that is important to measure. ΔG is defined by:

$$\Delta G = \Delta H - T \Delta S \qquad (3)$$

where Δ means the change, G is free energy, H is heat energy (also called enthalpy) of the system, T is the absolute temperature and S is the entropy of the system (see below). A chemical reaction can occur only if ΔG is negative.

Equation (3) was derived from the laws of thermodynamics, which were formulated to predict the directions of chemical reactions. There are several laws, but only some need concern us here.

Laws of thermodynamics

The **first law of thermodynamics** states that energy is conserved in a chemical system, i.e. the **total energy** of a system and its surroundings is a constant. The first law is in effect the conservation of energy. The energy may be converted from one form to another, for example from chemical bond energies to heat, and vice versa, but the total energy within the system is conserved. There is an equation derived from the first law:

$$\Delta E = E_2 - E_1 \qquad (4)$$

where ΔE is the energy change, E_2 is the energy of the system at the end of the reaction and E_1 is the energy at the start.

ΔE and ΔG are related by the equation:

$$\Delta G \approx \Delta E - T \Delta S \qquad (5)$$

The first law cannot predict if a reaction will occur spontaneously. For this, another law is summoned, namely the **second law of thermodynamics**, which states that a reaction can occur spontaneously only if there is a net increase in the sum of the **entropies** of the system and its surroundings.

Entropy is a term that means, quite simply, the degree of **disorder** or randomness of a system. An example of an increase in entropy is the diffusion of a solute such as a lump of sugar in a cup of tea. A negative entropy condition would be required to sustain the sugar in the hot tea as a lump. Similarly, negative entropy is a measure of the 'holding together' of biomolecules in their characteristic shape. Notice that ΔG gives no information about the **rate** of a reaction, only if it can occur spontaneously.

Types of reaction

In an **exothermic** reaction, heat is given off. Therefore, ΔH is negative. In an **endothermic** reaction, ΔH is positive since heat is absorbed by the system from its surroundings. According to the first law, no energy can be lost from the system during the chemical reaction, and in an **exergonic** reaction, the energy lost during the reaction is conserved as heat.

Standard free energy changes

Changes in free energy during a reaction are influenced by the pressure, temperature and the initial concentrations of the reactants and products. Biological reactions are also influenced by pH. In order to standardize free energy changes, standard conditions have been adopted: the temperature is taken to be 25°C (298 K); the pressure is 1 atm (1. 1325×10^5 Pa); the initial concentrations of reactants and products is 1 mol/l; the pH is taken as 7; the molar concentration of H_2O is taken as unity (1 mol/l). ΔG under these conditions is expressed as $\Delta G^{0\prime}$.

There is a formula for $\Delta G^{0\prime}$:

$$\Delta G = \Delta G^{0\prime} + R \log_e \frac{[C]\,[D]}{[A]\,[B]} \qquad (6)$$

where ΔG is the free energy change for a reaction, R is the gas constant, T is the absolute temperature and $\log_e$ is the natural logarithm.

From Equations (2) and (6), it can be worked out that:

$$\Delta G^{0\prime} = 2.303 \, RT \log_{10} K_{eq} \qquad (7)$$

Note: the **gas constant (R)** is also called the universal molar gas constant, and has a value of 8.134 J/mol per K. It means that all gases have the same kinetic energy for a fixed number of gas molecules and at a given temperature. The **absolute temperature** is measured in Kelvins (K). Theoretically, the lowest possible temperature is –273 K.

If K_{eq} is less than 1, $\Delta G^{0\prime}$ is positive. This means the reaction will not occur unless energy is applied. The reaction is said to be **endergonic**. If K_{eq} is greater than 1, the reaction will occur spontaneously because $\Delta G^{0\prime}$ is negative. The reaction is said to be **exergonic** (see above).

30 Chemical reactions II

OXIDATION–REDUCTION REACTIONS

Oxidation–reduction (**redox**) reactions are important in biochemistry and the mitochondrial electron transport chain, for example is better understood if the basic principles of redox reactions are known beforehand. Any substance that donates an electron to another in a chemical reaction is called a **reductant**. Any substance that accepts an electron is called an **oxidant**. Consider the equation:

$$2A^- + 2H^+ \rightarrow 2A + H_2 \tag{1}$$

which can also be written as two half-equations:

$$2A^- \rightarrow 2A + 2e^- \tag{2}$$

$$2H^+ + 2e^- \rightarrow H_2 \tag{3}$$

Compound A has been oxidized, and H^+ ions have been reduced to gaseous H_2.

Electron flow is part of electrochemical change, and is associated with an electromotive force (emf) that drives the reaction. This force can be measured, and is expressed as the **redox potential (E)**, and is a measure of the likelihood that a redox reaction will occur. E can be measured for reactions under standard conditions (1 atm of pressure; 298 K (25°C); pH 7) when it is termed E'_0 and expressed in volts.

Measurement of E'_0

E'_0 is measured as an electron flow between two half-cells, one of which is the sample cell, containing a solution of 1 mol/l concentration of the oxidant to be tested, linked by a bridge to a standard reference half-cell, which contains a 1 mol/1 solution of H^+ ions in equilibrium with H_2 gas at 1 atm. The voltage of the reference solution is taken as 0 V under these conditions. Electrons will flow from reductant to oxidant through electrodes immersed in the solution, and the emf is measured in a voltmeter.

> *Note*: although the potential of a standard H_2 electrode is set at 0 V, this is taken for pH = 0. When pH = 7.0, the E'_0 is –0.42 V.

Substance A in Equation (1) has a lower affinity for electrons than does H_2, and the E'_0 will be negative. A positive E'_0 means that the substance has a higher affinity for electrons than does H_2. A strong oxidizing agent, such as O_2, has a positive redox potential, while a strong reducing agent, such as nicotinamide adenine dinucleotide (NADH), has a negative redox potential.

The larger the positive E'_0, the stronger the oxidant, i.e. the higher is its affinity for electrons; in other words, it will tend to be reduced. The more negative the E'_0 is, the more easily will the reductant release electrons.

The tendency of the overall redox reaction to happen can be calculated simply by subtracting the redox potentials of the two half-reactions. For example, consider the exercise below.

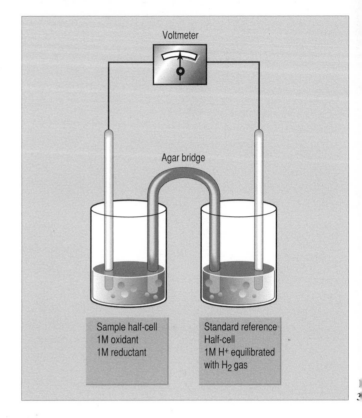

Voltmeter

Agar bridge

Sample half-cell
1M oxidant
1M reductant

Standard reference
Half-cell
1M H^+ equilibrated
with H_2 gas

Assume that we dissolve in 1 l of distilled H_2O, at 25°C, 1-g molecule (1 mol) of each of oxaloacetate, acetate, malate and acetaldehyde. Predict which substance will be oxidized, and which will be reduced. Which will be the oxidant and which the reductant?

$$\text{oxaloacetate} + 2H^+ + 2e^- \rightarrow \text{malate — where } E'_0 = -0.10 \text{ V} \tag{i}$$
$$\text{acetate} + 2H^+ + 2e^- \rightarrow \text{acetaldehyde — where } E'_0 = -0.60 \text{ V} \tag{ii}$$

Equation (i) has the more positive redox potential. Therefore, it will proceed more readily as a reduction, i.e. as it is written. Therefore, Equation (ii) will proceed in reverse as an oxidation.

Solving:

$$\text{oxaloacetate} + 2H^+ + 2e^- \rightarrow \text{malate}$$
$$\underline{\text{acetaldehyde} \rightarrow \text{acetate} + 2H^+ + 2e^-}$$
$$\text{oxaloacetate} + \text{acetaldehyde} \rightarrow \text{malate} + \text{acetate}$$

Oxaloacetate gains electrons and is reduced to malate, and acetaldehyde loses electrons and is oxidized to acetate. Therefore, acetaldehyde is the reducing agent, and oxaloacetate is the oxidizing agent.

Also:

$$\Delta E'_0 = (-0.10) - (-0.60) = -0.10 + 0.60$$
$$= +0.5 \text{ V}$$

FREE ENERGY OF OXIDATION

The free energy of oxidation, $\Delta G^{0\prime}$, is given by:

$$\Delta G^{0\prime} = -n\mathrm{F}\Delta E'_0 \tag{4}$$

where n is the number of electrons transferred per mole and F is the Faraday constant (96 500 J/V equiv.) Note that $\Delta E'_0$ must be positive in order for $\Delta G^{0\prime}$ to be negative.

THE NERNST EQUATION

The Nernst equation can be used to calculate the redox potential under non-standard conditions, in which the concentrations of the reactants are present at non-standard concentrations:

$$E = E_0 + \frac{RT}{n\mathrm{F}}\log_e \frac{[\text{oxidized form}]}{[\text{reduced form}]} \tag{5}$$

Expressed in terms of $\log_{10}$:

$$E = E_0 + \frac{2.303RT}{n\mathrm{F}}\log_{10} \frac{[\text{oxidized form}]}{[\text{reduced form}]} \tag{6}$$

Therefore, the Nernst equation can be expressed as:

$$E = E_0 + \frac{0.059}{n}\log_{10} \frac{[\text{oxidized form}]}{[\text{reduced form}]} \tag{7}$$

COUPLED REACTIONS

Biochemical reactions very often require energy; they may not 'go' by themselves, for example the formation of macromolecules such as nucleic acids and proteins from their respective nucleotide and amino acid subunits. This sort of elaboration requires work, which in turn requires energy. The energy is supplied by **exergonic** reactions. Exergonic reactions do the work that drive the **endergonic** reactions.

The cell has enzymes that catalyse exergonic reactions; some of the energy produced by the reactions is trapped by coupling the reaction to an endergonic reaction, which generates so-called **energy-rich compounds** such as ATP.

31 Enzymes I

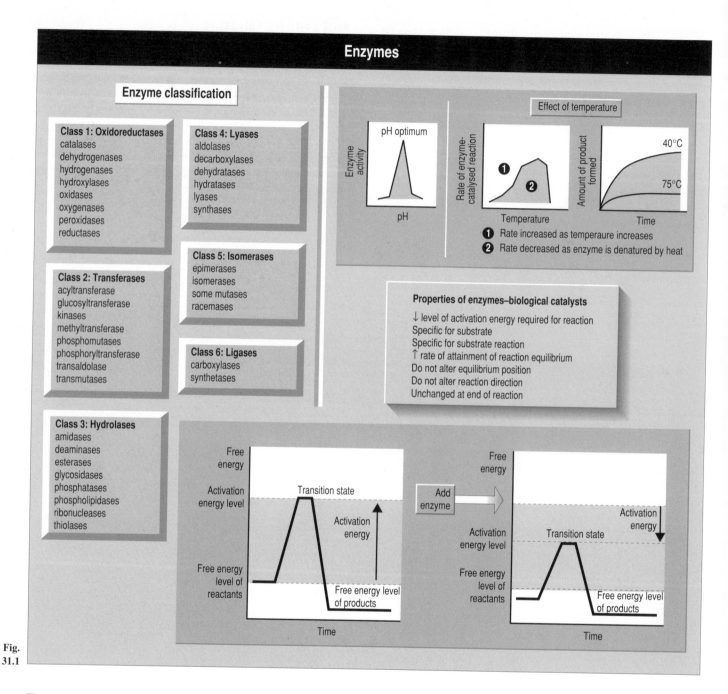

Fig. 31.1

Enzymes are proteins which catalyse chemical reactions. They can operate in the living cell, or in the test tube under the correct conditions, and are even put into washing powders for digesting food stains in clothing. Enzymes increase the rate at which a reaction reaches equilibrium, although they do not alter the thermodynamic properties of the reaction, for example the equilibruim constant of the reaction.

ACTIVATION STATES

Enzymes, like other catalysts, are not changed themselves after the reaction, although they may be temporarily altered in structure while the reaction is proceeding. Enzymes make reactions possible in the body, at rates which allow the cells to live. Normally, at 37°C and at a pH of 7, most of the reactions necessary for life would go too slowly.

During a chemical reaction, the reacting chemicals pass through an energy state higher than that of either the reactants or of the products. The reactants need to attain a certain **activation energy** in order to reach a so-called **transition state,** and the rate of the reaction will depend on the rate at which individual reacting molecules build up activation energy to the transition state.

Enzymes, like other catalysts, actually reduce the amount of activation energy required. They achieve this by providing alternative pathways for the reaction; these pathways require less activation energy than would be needed in the absence of the enzyme.

PROPERTIES OF ENZYMES

Substrate and reaction specificity

Unlike inorganic catalysts, such as platinum, which can catalyse a whole host of reactions in the test tube, the biological catalysts, the enzymes, are highly **specific**. They will recognize one or a few chemically closely related substrates. Substrates may be defined as substances on which enzymes act in biochemical reactions. Similarly, enzymes will catalyse specific **types** of reactions.

Chemical composition

Enzymes are macromolecules. They are almost all proteins (although it has been shown that RNA can catalyse certain reactions). They are composed of amino acid chains, whose specific sequences determine the folding, shape and function of the enzyme.

FACTORS AFFECTING ENZYME ACTIVITY

pH

The pH can affect biochemical reactions in a variety of ways:
1 extremes of pH may radically alter enzyme structure, and thus denature the enzyme;
2 the pH may affect the degree to which the substrate is ionized, and thus affect the rate of the reaction;
3 the pH can affect the binding of the enzyme and substrate;
4 the pH can alter the reactivity of the enzyme during the catalytic process.
Only (3) and (4) will be considered here.

Most enzymes are active only within a fairly limited pH range, and they have an optimum pH at which their activity is greatest. The pH optimum will depend on where in the organism the enzyme is physiologically active. For example, pepsin, a digestive enzyme, operates in the stomach in the presence of hydrochloric acid, and its pH optimum is around 2. Lysosomal enzymes have a pH optima of around 5, the pH in the lysosome.

Temperature

All chemical reactions are increased as the temprerature is increased, including enzyme-catalysed reactions. But, when enzymes are heated above 40°C many of them begin to become denatured, which results in a fall in activity and a fall in the rate of the reaction. Once the enzyme is denatured, comparatively little more of the product will be formed, no matter how long the reaction is left to proceed.

CLASSIFICATION OF ENZYMES

The Commission on Enzyme Nomenclature of the International Union of Biochemistry established a classification of enzymes into six classes.
1 Oxidoreductases: these catalyse oxidation–reduction reactions. An example is alcohol dehydrogenase, which oxidizes alcohol to acetaldehyde.
2 Transferases: these catalyse group transfer reactions. The groups transferred include methyl, ketone, nitrogenous or phosphorus groups. Examples of a transferase are hexokinase and methyl-transferase.
3 Hydrolases: these catalyse hydrolytic reactions. They cleave O–P, C–N and C–O bonds. Examples are the peptide hydrolases, which cleave peptide bonds.
4 Lyases: these catalyse the reversible addition of groups to double bonds, or formation of double bonds by removal of groups. For example, they may remove ammonia, CO_2 or H_2O during the reaction. An example is pyruvate decarboxylase, which decarboxylates a keto-acid to yield an aldehyde with release of CO_2.
5 Isomerases: these enzymes catalyse different kinds of isomerization, which involves the rearrangement of a molecule to yield one with different physical and/or chemical properties. There are different types of isomerase. The **epimerases** and **racemases** catalyse inversion at asymmetrical carbon atoms. For example, lactate racemase catalyses the conversion of L-lactate to D-lactate. The **mutases** catalyse the transfer of groups within a molecule. For example, phosphoglycerate mutase produces 3-phosphoglycerate from 2-phosphoglycerate.
6 Ligases: these are also termed synthetases. They catalyse the condensation of two molecules, and the reaction is coupled to the cleavage of a high-energy phosphate bond, such as is found in ATP. An example is pyruvate carboxylase, which condenses pyruvate and bicarbonate to yield oxaloacetate, which is coupled to the conversion of ATP to ADP.

32 Enzymes II

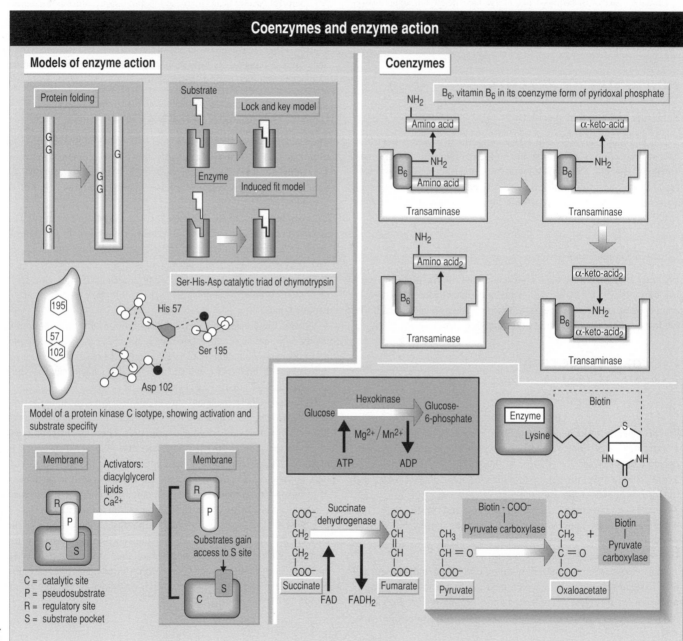

Fig. 32.1

MECHANISM OF ACTION

Protein folding

Enzymes are globular proteins consisting of one or more polypeptide chains which fold into a three-dimensional structure, depending on the amino acid sequence. The amino acids forming an active site may be far apart, but are brought into proximity through chain folding. Active sites on the enzyme surface include the substrate-binding, regulatory and catalytic sites. The nature and arrangement of the amino acids at a site determine, largely, the functional specificity of the active site.

Substrate–enzyme complex formation

The substrate is held at its binding site by non-covalent forces, including hydrogen and hydrophobic bonds, and electrostatic and van der Waals forces. The binding site is so specific for a substrate that often it will bind only one isomer of a diastereomeric pair. Some enzymes are not as specific. Glucokinase will bind only glucose, while hexokinase will bind and catalyse the phosphorylation of 2-deoxyglucose, fructose, glucosamine, glucose and mannose, although not all at the same rate.

It is believed that when the substrate makes contact with the active site, the site changes its conformation to accommodate the substrate. This is the **induced fit** model. Possibly, the induced fit mechanism places strains on the substrate, thereby lowering the activation energy required for the reaction to occur.

Mechanism of catalysis

The substrate-binding site is usually where some or all of the catalytic reaction occurs. **Chymotrypsin** is a digestive enzyme catalysing the hydrolysis of dietary proteins in the small intestine, cleaving peptide bonds at the carboxyl side of aromatic side chains of phenylalanine, tryptophan and tyrosine. There are two main steps in the reaction.
1 The substrate binds to the enzyme at a chemically active site dominated by a triad of three amino acids. These are Asp 102, His 57 and Ser 195, which form a **catalytic triad.** The substrate and the triad become bound by hydrogen bonding.
2 The susceptible peptide bond of the substrate is cleaved through the action of His 57 and Ser 195, and the peptide substrate is hydrolysed to yield an acid and an amine.

Regulatory sites on enzymes

Enzyme activity may be regulated by sites on the enzyme itself. Examples are enzymes that phosphorylate proteins, the **protein kinases.** Protein kinase C (PKC), a serine/threonine kinase, is activated by DAG, phospholipids and calcium ions, and is believed to mediate cellular events following activation of cells by hormones and second messengers. PKC appears to be a member of a family of PKC isotypes.

The enzyme has functionally distinct regions: a substrate pocket; an amino-terminal regulatory site; a pseudosubstrate site within the regulatory domain; and a carboxy-terminal catalytic site. The pseudosubstrate site consists of a sequence of amino acids resembling the substrate, but without a serine/threonine residue which can be phosphorylated. Instead, it contains an alanine residue. In the inactive state, the pseudosubstrate site occupies the substrate pocket within the catalytic domain and inactivates it. Activation of the enzyme causes a conformational change and dissociation of the pseudosubstrate from the substrate pocket. But, the pseudosubstrate still interacts with the substrate pocket, allowing only certain substrates to gain access to the pocket, thus playing a part in determining substrate specificity.

COFACTORS

Cofactors are chemicals that assist or are necessary for enzyme action. Cofactors become attached to the enzyme, usually at the catalytic site, and may enable the binding of the substrate and/or the catalytic process. There are two main groups: (i) **coenzymes;** and (ii) **prosthetic groups.**

Coenzymes

Coenzymes may be metals, e.g. cobalt, copper, iron, Mg^{2+}, manganese (Mn^{2+}) or Zn^{2+}. For example, Mg^{2+} or Mn^{2+} are needed for the reduction of the high negative charges of ATP during the kinase-catalysed phosphorylation reaction. The phosphorylation of glucose to glucose-6-phosphate provides an example of this type of reaction. Coenzymes may be organic molecules which are derived from vitamins.

Mechanism of coenzyme action. Coenzymes, such as flavine adenine dinucleotide (FAD) may be required as proton and electron acceptors. FAD is reduced to $FADH_2$ during dehydrogenation reactions, and in a separate reaction is oxidized back to FAD, which is ready to act as coenzyme again. Therefore, FAD is not only a coenzyme but a substrate too. Since the coenzyme is altered during the reaction, it is sometimes referred to as a **second substrate** for the enzyme.

Vitamin B_6 (pyridoxine) is an α-amino group acceptor which can transfer the δ-amino group to an α-keto-acid, thus forming a new amino acid.

Prosthetic groups

Prosthetic groups are non-proteins, which bind covalently to the enzyme at its active site. These include metal ions and organic molecules such as biotin. Biotin is vitamin B_4, and is required for the incorporation of CO_2 into organic compounds. It does this by acting as a carrier for CO_2.

Biotin binds covalently to a lysine residue at the catalytic site of the enzyme, and accepts $-COO^-$, usually from HCO_3^-. The $-COO^-$ is then passed rapidly to the substrate to form a carboxylated compound. Biotin needs ATP to bind CO_2.

Metals such as Zn^{2+} may function as cofactors by binding the substrate, and/or by promoting catalysis. Proteins that contain covalently bound metal ions are termed **metalloproteins.**

MULTISUBSTRATE REACTIONS

Enzyme reactions in which one enzyme may be able to bind more than one substrate may be **sequential** or what is sometimes called **'ping-pong'.** In a sequential reaction, one substrate may need to be bound before another, for example alcohol dehydrogenase first binds ethyl alcohol prior to binding the cofactor NAD^+. The reaction is said to be **ordered,** whereas one in which two substrates can bind in any order is said to be **random.** In a **ping-pong** reaction, an enzyme binds a substrate, converts it to a product which is released and then binds another substrate. An example is the transaminase reaction, where a keto-acid is released as product and another keto-acid bound as a substrate.

33 Enzymes III

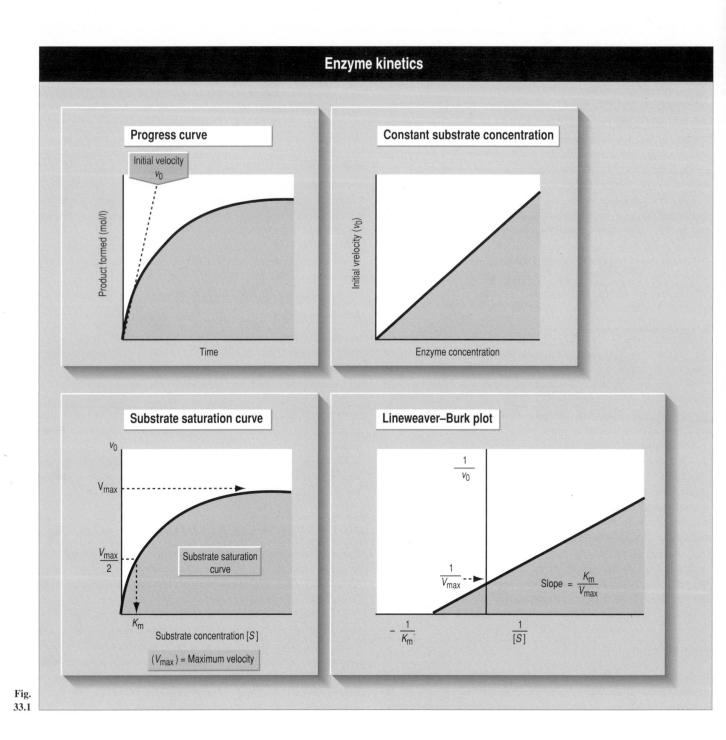

Fig. 33.1

ENZYME KINETICS

Enzyme–substrate interaction

When enzyme and substrate react together, the rate of the reaction will increase at first then slow down with time as the enzyme becomes degraded, or as equilibrium is approached. From the graph obtained, called a **progress curve**, we can derive the initial velocity, v_0. There is a direct relationship between v_0 and the enzyme concentration in the reaction mixture, in that the rate of the reaction will double when the enzyme concentration is doubled, for a given concentration of substrate.

Substrate saturation curve

If v_0 is plotted against substrate concentration at a given concentration of enzyme, then a curve is obtained whose shape we call a rectangular hyperbole. Initially, the rate of the reaction v_0 is directly proportional to the substrate concentration [S]. (Mathematicians call this 'first-order' kinetics.) But, as [S] increases, the rate eventually reaches a limiting maximum, V_{max}. The maximum reflects the fact that all the binding sites on the enzyme are taken up or saturated, and the rate could be increased only by adding more enzyme. This curve is called the **substrate saturation curve**. (Mathematicians call the 'bend' in the curve 'mixed' or first- and zero-order kinetics.) The flat part of the curve reflects the fact that there is no further increase in rate no matter how much substrate is added. (This is called 'zero-order' kinetics.)

Enzyme units

Enzyme activity is measured in units established by The Commission on Enzyme Nomenclature of the International Union of Biochemistry (SI). The unit is the **katal** (kat). One katal is the quantity of enzyme in the presence of which 1 mol of substrate is converted per second. It is more common, however, to express enzyme activity in millikatals or microkatals, since 1 kat is equivalent to the activity of about 1 kg of the pure enzyme. In many textbooks, enzyme activity is expressed as micromoles of substrate that are converted per minute to product under given assay conditions. The **standard unit** of enzyme activity, U, is the amount of enzyme catalysing the formation of 1 µmol of substrate per minute. The **specific activity** of an enzyme preparation is the number of enzyme units per milligram of protein. This gives an indication of the purity of the preparation.

The formula of the substrate saturation curve

The substrate saturation curve allows us to derive equilibrium constants that characterize the enzyme–substrate reaction for given conditions of pH and temperature. We can arbitrarily define a constant, the K_m, or **Michaelis constant**, which is the substrate concentration when the rate v_0 is half the maximum rate (see below). The equation that describes the curve was derived by Michaelis and Menten, and the equation they derived is called the **Michaelis–Menten equation**:

$$V_0 = \frac{V_{max}[S]}{K_m + [S]} \tag{1}$$

If v_0 is plotted against [S], a rectangular hyperbole is obtained. It is easy to calculate that when $v_0 = V_{max}/2$, then $K_m = [S]$.

In order to obtain values of K_m and V_{max}, the Michaelis–Menten equation can be linearized.

1 Invert Equation (1):

$$\frac{1}{v_0} = \frac{K_m + [S]}{V_{max}[S]} \tag{2}$$

2 Separate and simplify to give the Lineweaver–Burk plot:

$$\frac{1}{v_0} = \frac{K_m}{V_{max}} \cdot \frac{1}{[S]} + \frac{1}{V_{max}} \tag{3}$$

The Lineweaver–Burk plot is the equation of a straight line ($y = mx + c$), when $1/v_0$ (y) is plotted against $1/[S]$ (x), with gradient (m) = K_m/V_{max}, and the intercept (c) on the ordinate is $1/V_{max}$. $1/K_m$ can be read directly from the graph where the line crosses the abscissa.

Although not presented here, there are other methods of linearizing the Michaelis–Menten equation, which are generally favoured by biochemists.

34 Enzymes IV

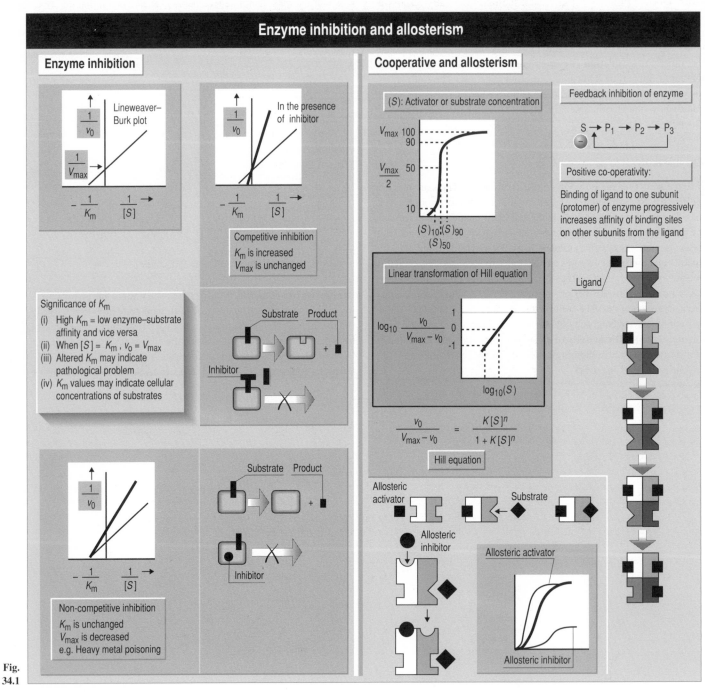

Enzyme inhibition and allosterism

Enzyme inhibition

Lineweaver–Burk plot

$\frac{1}{v_0}$

$\frac{1}{V_{max}}$

$-\frac{1}{K_m}$ $\frac{1}{[S]}$

In the presence of inhibitor

$\frac{1}{v_0}$

$-\frac{1}{K_m}$ $\frac{1}{[S]}$

Competitive inhibition
K_m is increased
V_{max} is unchanged

Significance of K_m
(i)   High K_m = low enzyme–substrate affinity and vice versa
(ii) When $[S] = K_m$, $v_0 = V_{max}$
(iii) Altered K_m may indicate pathological problem
(iv) K_m values may indicate cellular concentrations of substrates

Substrate   Product

Inhibitor

$\frac{1}{v_0}$

$-\frac{1}{K_m}$ $\frac{1}{[S]}$

Non-competitive inhibition
K_m is unchanged
V_{max} is decreased
e.g. Heavy metal poisoning

Substrate   Product

Inhibitor

Cooperative and allosterism

(S): Activator or substrate concentration

V_{max} 100
90
$\frac{V_{max}}{2}$ 50
10

$(S)_{10}$ $(S)_{90}$
$(S)_{50}$

Linear transformation of Hill equation

$\log_{10} \frac{v_0}{V_{max} - v_0}$

1
0
-1

$\log_{10}(S)$

$$\frac{v_0}{V_{max} - v_0} = \frac{K[S]^n}{1 + K[S]^n}$$

Hill equation

Allosteric activator   Substrate

Allosteric inhibitor

Allosteric activator

Allosteric inhibitor

Feedback inhibition of enzyme

$S \rightarrow P_1 \rightarrow P_2 \rightarrow P_3$

Positive co-operativity:

Binding of ligand to one subunit (protomer) of enzyme progressively increases affinity of binding sites on other subunits from the ligand

Ligand

Fig. 34.1

KINETICS OF ENZYME INHIBITION

Enzymes may be inhibited from acting by small ions or molecules which form part of regulatory control systems or by drugs. Inhibition of enzyme action may be **irreversible** or **reversible**. Reversible inhibition may be **competitive** or **non-competitive**; the nature of reversible inhibition can be determined using enzyme kinetics and the Lineweaver–Burk plot. Some small molecules may control enzyme activity by binding to **allosteric sites**, which inhibit or activate the enzyme. Many enzymes are **oligomers**, being formed of identical subunits or **protomers**, each with a substrate-binding site. Activation of an allosteric site on one protomer may increase substrate–enzyme affinity on other protomers, a process called **co-operativity**.

Irreversible inhibition

Irreversible inhibition is permanent enzyme inhibition, usually due to the covalent attachment of a chemical to the enzyme at one or more of its active sites, or at another site which alters the conformational shape of the enzyme. The organism has to produce more enzyme to replace it. Examples of irreversible inhibitors are heavy metal ions such as mercury ions. Nerve gases such as the organophosphorus compound di-isopropylphosphofluoridate (DFP) bind irreversibly to the specific serine in the active centre of a large group of hydrolases, for example acetylcholinesterase.

Reversible inhibitors

Reversible inhibitors bind to enzymes non-covalently and are able to dissociate, thus leaving them free to catalyse substrates. Reversible inhibitors can be removed by dialysis.

Competitive inhibition

A competitive inhibitor competes with the substrate for its binding site on the enzyme, and is often structurally similar to the substrate. Once bound, the inhibitor may itself be converted to a product, or occupy the site until it dissociates from it. The action of the inhibitor can be overcome by increasing the concentration of the normal substrate at the binding site. The Lineweaver–Burk plot in the presence of a fixed concentration of the inhibitor reflects competitive inhibition through an apparent increase in the K_m, and an unaltered V_{max}.

An example of a competitive inhibitor is malonate, which competes with succinate at its binding site on the enzyme succinate dehydrogenase, where succinate is normally converted to fumarate. If the concentration of succinate is increased, it will displace malonate from the enzyme. Examples of metabolized inhibitors are the antibiotic sulphonamides, such as **sulphanilamide**, which bind to dihydropterate synthetase, a bacterial enzyme that synthesizes folic acid from p-aminobenzoate, which is necessary for bacterial growth. The enzyme converts the sulphonamide to a compound that cannot be metabolized to folic acid, and the bacteria die.

Non-competitive inhibition

Non-competitive inhibitors usually bind to the enzyme at sites other than that which binds the substrate, and the substrate does not compete with the inhibitor. Therefore, although the substrate may still be able to occupy its own binding site on the enzyme, it is not converted to product. The inhibitor–enzyme–substrate complex is sometimes called a 'dead-end' complex, since it is catalytically inactive. Non-competitive inhibitors in effect remove enzyme from the available pool, and the Lineweaver–Burk plot reflects this in that the K_m is unchanged but the V_{max} is reduced.

ALLOSTERISM

Allosterism is a word used to describe enzymes that have binding sites for molecules, usually of low molecular weight, other than those where substrates bind and are converted to product. These small molecules are termed **ligands**. A ligand is a molecule that binds to a binding site on a macromolecule, such as an enzyme or a receptor. These allosteric binding sites are very often where enzyme activity is controlled. Ligands that bind to allosteric binding sites may be **allosteric activators** or **allosteric inhibitors**. The product of an enzyme may itself be an allosteric inhibitor, binding to and inhibiting an enzyme further back in the chain of metabolic pathways that produced it. This is an example of a physiological control mechanism whereby metabolic processes are regulated.

Classes of allosteric enzymes

Allosteric enzymes have been classified as **K class** and **V class**, depending on how their allosteric ligands affect the kinetic constants K_m and V_{max}. In the presence of their allosteric ligands, K-class enzymes yield plots showing an altered K_m and unchanged V_{max} (as is seen with competitive inhibitors of enzyme action). In other words, an allosteric inhibitor binds to the allosteric site, and the enzyme reacts by losing affinity for the substrate.

In the presence of their allosteric inhibitors, V-class enzymes yield plots showing an unchanged K_m and lower V_{max} (as is seen with non-competitive enzyme inhibitors).

Mechanism of allosterism

The mechanism of allosterism is not well understood, but it is believed that when a ligand binds to an allosteric site it alters the conformation of the enzyme so that the affinity of the substrate (or some other ligand) for its binding site on the enzyme is either increased or decreased, depending on whether the ligand is an allosteric activator or inhibitor, respectively.

If a ligand increases the affinity of another protomer for the same ligand, this is termed a **homotrophic** interaction. If the ligand increases the affinity of another protomer for a different ligand, this is termed a **heterotrophic** interaction.

Co-operativity is the term used to describe the effect that one protomer can exert on another, as happens when a ligand binds. Co-operativity reveals itself in the substrate saturation curve, which is sigmoidal, and the formula of the line is given by the **Hill equation**, which can be linearized. Allosteric activators will shift the curve to the left, while inhibitors will shift the curve to the right. The binding of O_2 to Hb provides another example of positive co-operativity and a sigmoidal curve. Note, however, that sigmoidal curves will always be obtained with multisubunit enzymes, even in the absence of co-operativity.

Allosteric effects can occur on one protomer **without** a co-operative effect on other protomers. For example, alcohol dehydrogenase is a zinc-containing metalloprotein which reduces acetaldehyde to alcohol, and consists of protomers which are independently activated allosterically.

35 Digestion: basic principles and cell types

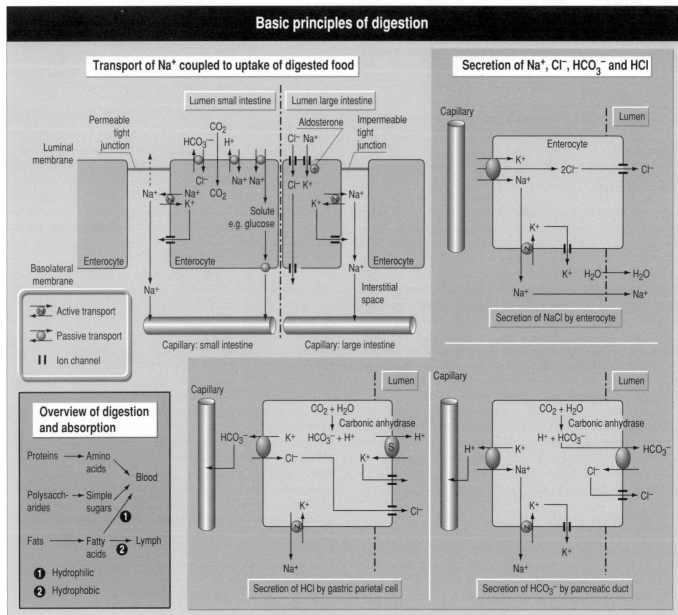

Basic principles of digestion

Transport of Na+ coupled to uptake of digested food

Secretion of Na+, Cl−, HCO3− and HCl

Overview of digestion and absorption

Fig. 35.1

INTRODUCTION

When food is ingested, it is not in a form that can be readily absorbed by the cells of the alimentary tract. For efficient absorption to occur, the polymeric foodstuffs are hydrolysed into their constitutive residues, which can be taken up more easily into the epithelial cells.

Digestive enzymes are released in controlled secretions from specialized organs and cells of the alimentary tract. These secretions also contain compositions of solutes to maximize the activity of the enzymes. Daily, 1–2 l of saliva are secreted into the mouth, 2.5 l of gastric juice are secreted into the stomach, 1–3 l are secreted into the small intestine by the epithelial cells of the intestinal wall and 1 l of bile and 1 l of pancreatic juice drain directly into the duodenum.

Due to the differences in the composition of the secretions, the pH of the tract varies widely. In the stomach, the pH is usually 4.0 due to the secretion of hydrochloric acid, but in the duodenum the pH rises to 6.5–6.8 with the addition of bicarbonate ions in the pancreatic juice.

The epithelial cells of the intestinal wall, therefore, are not only adapted to the absorption of digested foods but also to the maintenance of a luminal environment in which digestion and absorption can occur at maximal rates.

Solute transport

There are two distinct pathways for solute transport: (i) the solutes may pass through the tight junctions which connect the epithelial cells of the intestinal wall to each other (**paracellular route**); or (ii) they may pass directly through the epithelial cells themselves, so passing through the luminal membrane and the basolateral membrane (**transcellular route**).

The luminal membrane contains many protein transport molecules that are specialized for uptake or secretion of solutes and of digestive enzymes. The basolateral membrane is more typical of the plasma membrane of most cells, while also showing transport systems for the exit of nutrients absorbed into the cell from the lumen.

The dominant driving force for almost all of the transcellular solute movement against an electrochemical gradient is the Na^+/K^+–ATPase in the basolateral membrane. The actions of this energy-consuming transport protein are responsible for low Na^+ and high K^+ concentrations in the cytosol and an electrical potential of the cytoplasm of -60 mV compared with the extracellular fluid. The potential difference is caused by the asymmetrical transport of the ions by the protein (three Na^+ ions are transported out, while two K^+ ions are transported in).

MECHANISMS FOR THE ABSORBTION OF SOLUTES

The Na^+ in the lumen of the small and large intestines orginates from both the dietary intake and the secretions of the exocrine glands which drain into the intestinal tract. The uptake of Na^+ into the enterocytes along with Cl^- is therefore crucial to the maintenance of overall electrolyte balance in the body. The transport of Na^+ is also intimately involved in the uptake of digested food molecules such as glucose and amino acids (see Fig. 35.1).

The tight junctions connecting the epithelial cells in the large intestine are much less permeable to Na^+ and H_2O than are those in the small intestine. This correlates with the Na^+-scavenging function of the large intestine and the ability of the small intestine to secrete Na^+.

Uptake of solutes

The **luminal transporter** involves the uptake of solutes such as glucose or amino acids: Na^+ flows into the cell down the electrochemical gradient, established by the Na^+/K^+–ATPase, through a cotransport protein which carries the solute across the luminal membrane against its concentration gradient. This cotransporter can transport both ways, but is influenced in one direction by the negative potential in the cell.

In the small intestine, six specific carrier-mediated cotransporter systems for L-amino acids have been identified: (i) acidic amino acids, e.g. aspartate; (ii) basic amino acids, e.g. arginine; (iii) uncharged amino acids with polar or short side chains, e.g. threonine; (iv) uncharged amino acids with hydrophobic or aromatic side chains, e.g. methionine; (v) imino acids, e.g. proline; and (vi) β-amino acids, e.g. taurine.

D-fructose, D-glucose and D-galactose are the main monosaccharides resulting from digestion of carbohydrates. The latter two are absorbed by a monosaccharide cotransporter on the luminal membrane as described above, while D-fructose is absorbed through the luminal membrane by a facilitated diffusion mechanism which is Na^+ independent.

The **basolateral transporter** is a different type of transport system which facilitates the passage of the absorbed solute from the epithelial cell into the bloodstream. The basolateral transporter is not a cotransporter.

MECHANISMS FOR THE SECRETION OF SOLUTES

The secretion of solutes other than the digestive enzymes themselves is important for a number of reasons.

1 The changes in osmotic pressure that result from the movement of the solutes from the epithelial cell layer cause the movement of H_2O into the lumen of the tract. The H_2O is necessary to provide a more effective medium for digestion.

2 Enzymes in different areas of the digestive tract require differing conditions for their maximal efficiency, and the controlled secretion of acidic and basic ions can provide the enzymes with the environment that they need.

Na^+ and Cl^- can be secreted by most of the epithelial cells of the intestinal tract, but the pH of lumen is controlled by specialized cell types that secrete bicarbonate ions into the pancreatic juice and hydrochloric acid into the stomach.

PATHOPHYSIOLOGY

Vibrio cholerae is an infection of the gastrointestinal tract. Toxins that are produced by the bacteria cause excessive secretion of electrolytes by the stimulation of a cAMP regulatory pathway. The resulting diarrhoea can be life-threatening due to loss of essential electrolytes and H_2O. Treatment is based on the fact that the Na^+–glucose cotransporter is not regulated by a cAMP pathway and so administration of oral glucose will cause absorption of Na^+.

36 Digestion of protein and carbohydrates

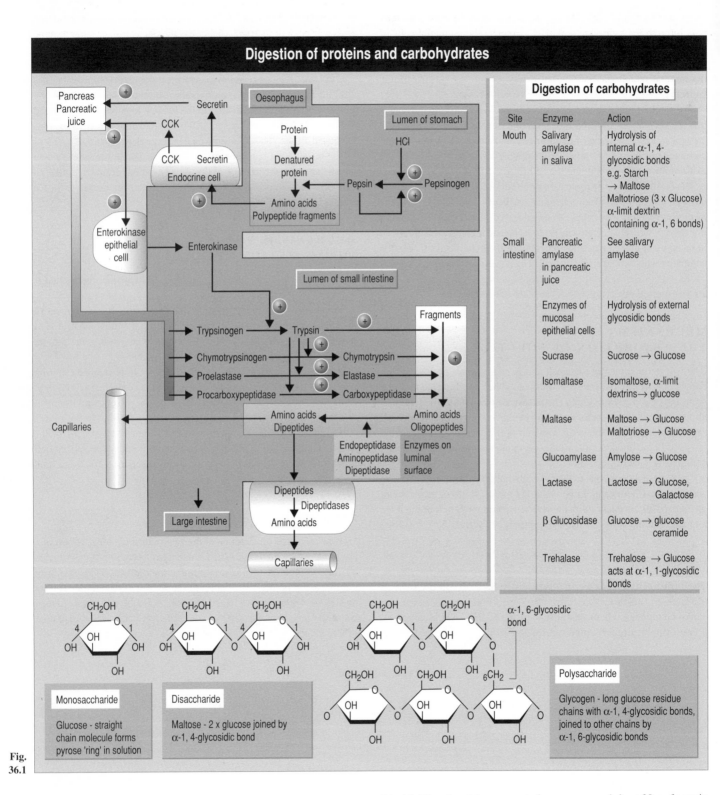

Digestion of proteins and carbohydrates

Digestion of carbohydrates

Site	Enzyme	Action
Mouth	Salivary amylase in saliva	Hydrolysis of internal α-1, 4-glycosidic bonds e.g. Starch $\rightarrow$ Maltose Maltotriose (3 x Glucose) α-limit dextrin (containing α-1, 6 bonds)
Small intestine	Pancreatic amylase in pancreatic juice	See salivary amylase
	Enzymes of mucosal epithelial cells	Hydrolysis of external glycosidic bonds
	Sucrase	Sucrose $\rightarrow$ Glucose
	Isomaltase	Isomaltose, α-limit dextrins $\rightarrow$ glucose
	Maltase	Maltose $\rightarrow$ Glucose Maltotriose $\rightarrow$ Glucose
	Glucoamylase	Amylose $\rightarrow$ Glucose
	Lactase	Lactose $\rightarrow$ Glucose, Galactose
	β Glucosidase	Glucose $\rightarrow$ glucose ceramide
	Trehalase	Trehalose $\rightarrow$ Glucose acts at α-1, 1-glycosidic bonds

Monosaccharide

Glucose - straight chain molecule forms pyrose 'ring' in solution

Disaccharide

Maltose - 2 x glucose joined by α-1, 4-glycosidic bond

Polysaccharide

Glycogen - long glucose residue chains with α-1, 4-glycosidic bonds, joined to other chains by α-1, 6-glycosidic bonds

Fig. 36.1

DIGESTION OF PROTEINS

On average, a 70-kg man eats 80–100 g of protein daily. In addition to this, 10–20 g of protein are secreted as enzymes and about 20 g of protein as mucosal cells that are sloughed off from the intestinal surface into the lumen of the intestine. Virtually all of this protein is digested and absorbed.

The first stage of protein digestion occurs in the mouth with the mechanical breakdown of the food by the teeth. This provides a larger surface area for the later stages.

Protein digestion in the stomach

In the stomach, hydrochloric acid secreted by the parietal cells kills invading bacteria and causes unravelling of the protein chains or **denaturation**, providing an increased surface area for digestion. The first stage of enzymatic digestion also occurs in the stomach. When digestive enzymes are released into the lumen, they are in an inactive form (**zymogens**) so that they will not damage the mucosal surfaces of the epithelial cells that line the intestine. **Pepsinogen** is released by zymogen-releasing cells in the stomach, and is the precursor for the digestive enzyme **pepsin**. Cleavage of the peptide bond between residues 44 and 45 of pepsinogen to release pepsin can occur spontaneously at a pH more acidic than 5 (as provided by the hydrochloric acid (**auto-activation**)), or by active cleavage of the peptide bond by pepsin itself (**autocatalysis**). Pepsin is stable only in the acidic environment of the stomach and cleaves peptide bonds on the $-NH_2$ side of aromatic amino acids, e.g. tyrosine (Tyr), phenylalanine (Phe). The large peptide fragments and amino acids which result stimulate secretion of digestive enzymes into the small intestine.

Digestion of proteins in the small intestine

Digestion of proteins in the small intestine is triggered by the controlled release of **enterokinase** from duodenal epithelial cells, and is dependent on the release of bicarbonate ions, which neutralize the acid from the stomach. Enterokinase cleaves a hexapeptide from **trypsinogen**, one of the zymogens released from the pancreas, to form **trypsin**. Trypsin, in addition to its own autocatalytic powers, cleaves peptide fragments off other pancreatic zymogens to activate them. The activated pancreatic enzymes hydrolyse peptide bonds at different sites along the polypeptide chains. There are two carboxypeptidases that release amino acids from the carboxyl terminal of the protein. Trypsin, **chymotrypsin** and **elastase** are endopeptidases and will digest the protein from within the chain.

Oligopeptides resulting from the action of the pancreatic enzymes are further digested by endopeptidases, aminopeptidases and dipeptidases present on the luminal surface of epithelial cells of the intestine. The final products of the luminal digestion are amino acids, dipeptides and tripeptides, which can be taken up into the epithelial cells. Further hydrolysis of peptide bonds occurs in the epithelial cells before the final transport of amino acids into the portal blood. In general, all dipeptides and tripeptides are broken down into their constituent amino acids in the epithelial cell. Exceptions to this rule include peptides that contain proline, hydroxyproline or unusual amino acids.

DIGESTION OF CARBOHYDRATES

Nature of carbohydrates

The three most common carbohydrate products of digestion, **glucose**, **galactose** and **fructose** are all examples of hexose monosaccharides. Monosaccharides are the simplest form of carbohydrates as they are comprised of one sugar unit, which is the basis for the structure of more complex carbohydrates. Disaccharides contain two sugar units, oligosaccharides contain a few units and polysaccharides contain many units. The general formula for monosaccharides is $C_nH_{2n}O_n$. The simplest monosaccharides contain three carbon atoms. Those containing four, five, six or seven carbons are called tetroses, pentoses, hexoses or heptoses, respectively. The carbon atoms in the monosaccharide are numbered so that an aldehyde or keto group is at the low number end and a primary alcohol is at the high number end. Almost all the carbohydrates in the body exist in the R–configuration. This refers to the configuration of atoms around C_{n-1}, which determines whether a R-isomer or a S-isomer is formed. Two further isomers are formed when a monosaccharide forms a ring structure in solution: α- and β-isomers. α and β refer to the arrangement of the –H and –OH groups around C_1.

The bond that connects sugar units to each other is called a glycosidic bond, and when formed between two monosaccharides involves the loss of H_2O, i.e. it is a condensation reaction.

Carbohydrates are stored in the form of long-chain polysaccharides whose units are joined by glycosidic bonds. The existence of long chains of units avoids the generation of osmotic pressures in a cell, which would occur with the equivalent number of units stored separately or in smaller chains. Glycogen is the major storage form of carbohydrates in animals. In plants, the equivalent storage molecule is **starch**. Starch is made up of **amylopectin**, which has the same structure as glycogen except that the branch points are less common, and amylose which is made up of glucose residues joined by α-1,4-glycosidic links and has no branch points.

The dietary carbohydrates are made up mainly of starch, sucrose and lactose. In the mouth, the efficiency of the salivary amylase is limited by the extent that the food has been chewed. Acid in the stomach inactivates salivary amylase, but may hydrolyse some of the glycosidic bonds.

PATHOPHYSIOLOGY

Lactase deficiency or milk intolerance is the most frequent of the disaccharidase deficiency syndromes. The inability to digest lactose in the upper small intestine results in bacterial fermentation of the sugar in the lower small intestine. The products of the fermentation include gas, which causes abdominal distension and flatulence, and osmotically active solutes which cause diarrhoea. Treatment includes prior digestion of the milk by commercially purified lactase.

37 Digestion and absorption of lipids

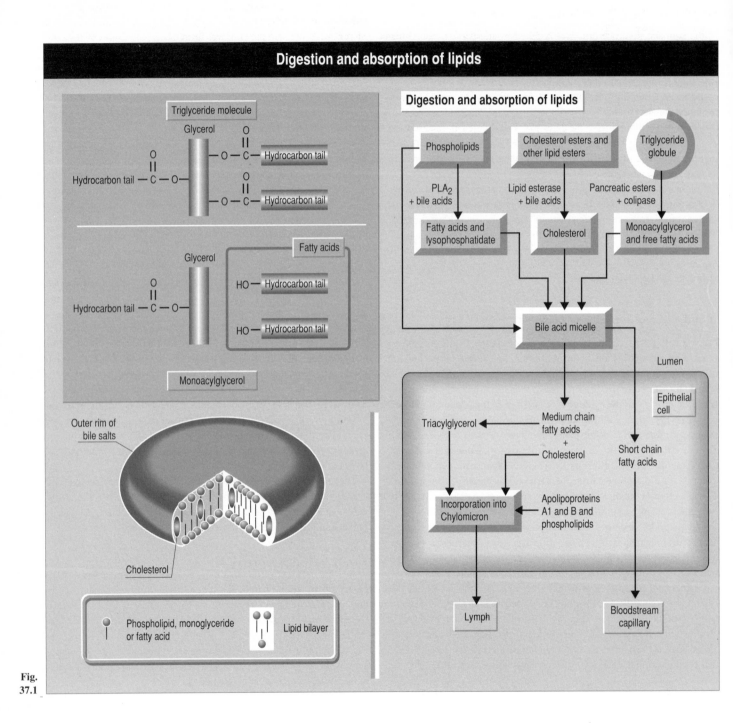

Digestion and absorption of lipids

Fig. 37.1

INTRODUCTION

Lipids (or fats) are found in nuts, cheese, milk and oils, and their daily intake in a healthy normal adult is between 60 and 150 g. Most of this is in the form of **triacylglycerols (triglycerides)**. Phospholipids, cholesterol, cholesterol esters and free fatty acids are also present.

Triglycerides and fatty acids

Triglycerides are the most common form of lipid and they are composed of three fatty acids joined by an ester linkage to a molecule of glycerol. Fatty acids are characterized by a long hydrocarbon tail with a carboxyl tail. The most common length for these is between 16 and 18 carbon molecules, although lengths may range from four up to

24 molecules. Each fatty acid has a carboxyl and a methyl terminal. The carbon atom that comprises the carboxyl terminal is numbered C_1. The adjacent carbon is numbered C_2, but is also known as the α-carbon. The carbon that comprises the methyl terminal is known as the ω-carbon.

DIGESTION OF LIPIDS

Lipids are hydrophobic in nature and in an aqueous solution are insoluble and aggregate together. This applies to both the digestive substrates and also to most of the products. The result is that a comparatively large volume of lipids has a small surface area. The digestive process acts to: (i) increase the surface area of lipids; and (ii) 'solubilize' the digestive products so that they can be absorbed.

Gastric digestion

Digestion of lipids begins in the stomach with the action of **lingual lipase**. This is released by glands at the back of the tongue and is active at the acidic pH of the stomach. The action of the lipase is to hydrolyse triglyceride molecules to form free fatty acids, monoacylglycerols, diacylglycerols and glycerol. The action of gastric lipase is aided by churning movements of the stomach, which act to disperse the lipids into a fine emulsion increasing the surface area for digestion.

Intestinal digestion

The main part of the digestion of the fats occurs in the small intestine and is co-ordinated by components of both the pancreatic juice (bicarbonate ions and enzymes) and bile (bile acids). Bicarbonate ions from the pancreatic juice neutralize the acid from the stomach and provide optimal pH conditions for the digestive enzymes. These include pancreatic lipase, lipid esterase and phospholipase A_2, all of which are secreted from the pancreas. **Pancreatic lipase** has the same action as the gastric lipase, but preferentially acts on lipids whose fatty acids contain over 10 atoms of carbon. The enzyme shows inhibition by bile acids but this is overcome by **colipase**, which binds to and activates lipase while holding it to the H_2O–lipid interface. Colipase is secreted by the pancreas as procolipase and is activated by hydrolysis at its amino terminal by trypsin. **Lipid esterase** hydrolyses most lipid esters, e.g. cholesterol esters and monoglycerides, and **phospholipase A_2** hydrolyses phospholipids. Both the lipid esterase and the phospholipase A_2 require bile acids for efficient function.

Bile salts. Bile salts are synthesized in the liver from cholesterol and are released into the duodenum where they aid the digestion and absorption of fats. The bile salts are amphipathic molecules and in solution aggregate to form a **micelle** with the hydrophilic parts of the salts facing the solution, while the hydrophobic parts of the salts face inward. Free fatty acids and monoacylglycerols are slightly more H_2O-soluble than are lipids, and as they equilibrate with the aqueous surroundings they will be incorporated into the bile salt micelle. Cholesterol and phospholipids are also incorporated into the micelle.

ABSORPTION OF FAT

The bile salt micelles transport their contents to the wall of the small intestine and so concentrate the digested fats next to the cells into which they are to be absorbed. The contents of the luminal area adjacent to these cells are very poorly mixed and without the micelles the digested fats would not be able to achieve the steep concentration gradients that are necessary for efficient absorption into the epithelial cells. The absorption of fats occurs mostly in the jejunum, whereas the absorption of bile acids occurs via a Na^+–bile salt cotransport system in the ileum. The salts then pass to the liver where they are recycled.

Inside the cells, the fate of fatty acids depends on the length of their hydrocarbon tail. Fatty acids whose tails are less than 12 carbon atoms long, pass directly into the bloodstream. Fatty acids whose tails are over 12 carbon atoms are conjugated to a binding protein and transported to the smooth ER. Here, they are incorporated into triglycerides which form lipid globules. Modification in the ER and Golgi apparatus results in the formation of specific lipoproteins called chylomicrons.

Transport of absorbed lipids: the exogenous pathway

Chylomicrons in the epithelial cells pass into the intestinal lymph vessels. These lead ultimately to the thoracic duct which empties into the left subclavian vein. This blood passes through the lungs before reaching the capillaries of the peripheral tissues.

Most of the chylomicron constituents are taken up by peripheral tissues, especially adipose and muscle tissues. At the surface of these tissues the triglycerides are hydrolysed by lipoprotein lipase; the fatty acids are then taken up and reassembled into triglycerides inside the cell. The lipoprotein that remains after depletion of most of the chylomicron is a chylomicron remnant and is taken up in the liver by receptor-mediated endocytosis.

PATHOPHYSIOLOGY

Cholesterol and phospholipids are secreted in equal proportions by the liver into the bile. It is important that there are equal proportions of cholesterol and phospholipids because cholesterol is insoluble in aqueous solution and the two are only solubilized in the bile by their incorporation into a bile acid/phospholipid micelle. When too much cholesterol is secreted into the bile, it precipitates out of solution to form crystals. **Gallstones** can eventually form from the crystals and these may become lodged in the cystic duct, causing abdominal pain, vomiting, steatorrhoea and jaundice.

38 The production of energy in the electron transfer chain

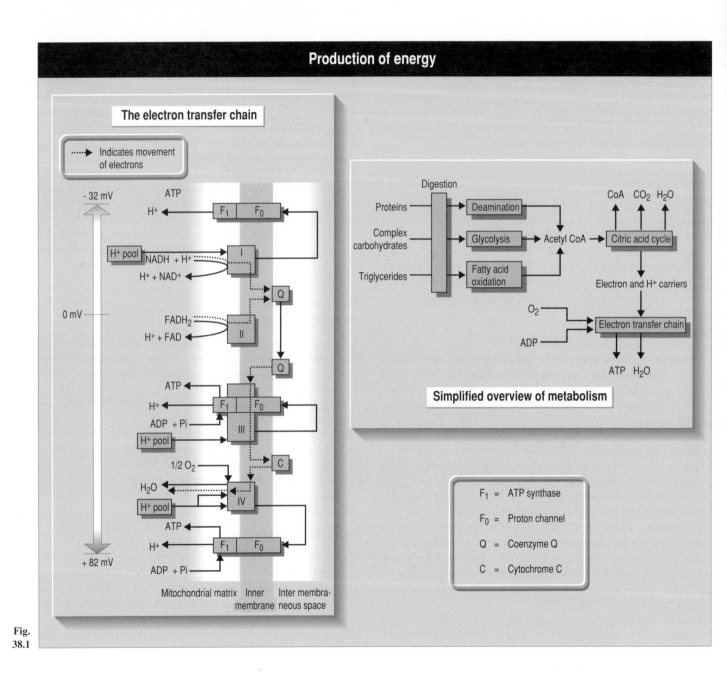

Production of energy

The electron transfer chain

······▶ Indicates movement of electrons

- 32 mV

0 mV

+ 82 mV

ATP

H^+

F_1 F_0

H^+ pool NADH + H^+

H^+ + NAD^+

I

Q

$FADH_2$

H^+ + FAD

II

Q

ATP

H^+

ADP + Pi

H^+ pool

III

$1/2$ O_2

H_2O

H^+ pool

IV

C

ATP

H^+

ADP + Pi

F_1 F_0

Mitochondrial matrix Inner membrane Inter membraneous space

Simplified overview of metabolism

Digestion

Proteins → Deamination

Complex carbohydrates → Glycolysis → Acetyl CoA

Triglycerides → Fatty acid oxidation

CoA CO_2 H_2O

Citric acid cycle

Electron and H^+ carriers

O_2

ADP

Electron transfer chain

ATP H_2O

F_1 = ATP synthase

F_0 = Proton channel

Q = Coenzyme Q

C = Cytochrome C

Fig. 38.1

INTRODUCTION

When foodstuffs are digested they are broken down into units that are less complex than their parent compounds. Polysaccharides are broken down into monosaccharides such as glucose, proteins into amino acids and fats into glycerol and fatty acids. Digestion can be thought of as the first stage of energy generation. As this is achieved, the potential energy that is 'contained' in the food molecules is transferred into a form which can be used by the body to fuel its various energy-requiring activities.

COUPLING OF REACTIONS TO THE HYDROLYSIS OF ATP

This principle of coupling reactions is used extensively in biological processes, and one of the main forms of energy currency is **ATP**. The $\Delta G^{0'}$ for the hydrolysis of ATP is –37 kJ/mol and the products of the reaction are ADP and Pi (see below). Under the conditions that exist intracellularly, the actual change in free energy that accompanies the hydrolysis of ATP is closer to –60 kJ/mol.

$$ATP^{4-} + H_2O \rightarrow ADP^{3-} + Pi^{2-} + H^+$$

The free energy that is released by the hydrolysis of ATP is used to fuel four types of activities in the body: (i) synthesis of macromolecules; (ii) active transport of ions; (iii) thermogenesis; and (iv) contraction of muscles. Hydrolysis of other phosphorylated nucleotides is also used to provide energy for endergonic reactions, but not to the extent that ATP is used. For example, cytosine triphosphate is hydrolysed to fuel synthesis of phospholipids.

PHOSPHATE TRANSFER POTENTIAL

The ability of a molecule to release free energy with the hydrolytic removal of a phosphate group is known as its **phosphate transfer potential**. Of the phosphorylated molecules involved in metabolism the phosphate transfer potential of ATP occupies a relatively intermediate position. Hydrolysis of the phosphate group of phosphoenolpyruvate has a $\Delta G^{0'}$ of -62 kJ/mol, while that of glucose-1-phosphate is only -14 kJ/mol. It follows, therefore, that hydrolysis of phosphoenolpyruvate can provide enough free energy to phosphorylate ADP to form ATP, while hydrolysis of glucose-1-phosphate cannot. The formation of ATP from ADP is important as there is only a limited quantity of the nucleotide in the body and almost all the cells in the body can phosphorylate ADP.

THE ELECTRON TRANSFER CHAIN

It is the controlled metabolism of digested food molecules that is responsible for the synthesis of ATP. This involves the oxidation of the digested products to CO_2 and H_2O, and involves a large number of reaction-specific enzymes. The oxidative reactions of metabolism all involve the transfer of two molecules of hydrogen (H^+) and two electrons (e^-) from one metabolite to another. The metabolite that loses the two H^+ and the two e^- is then said to be oxidized while the receiving metabolite is said to be reduced and the two make up a redox couple. The principles of redox potential and redox coupling have been discussed in Chapter 30.

In metabolism, when two H^+ and two e^- are removed from a substrate by a dehydrogenase enzyme, they are passed onto a coenzyme. There are three coenzymes that are involved in oxidative processes: **nicotinamide adenine dinucleotide (NAD^+)** and **flavine adenine dinucleotide (FAD^+)** which are involved in the synthesis of ATP, and **nicotinamide adenine dinucleotide phosphate ($NADP^+$)**, which is involved in the synthesis of macromolecules.

$$NAD(P)^+ + 2H^+ + 2e^- \rightarrow NAD(P)H + H^+$$
$$FAD + 2H^+ + 2e^- \rightarrow FADH_2$$

NAD^+ and $NADP^+$ are able to move freely between different dehydrogenase enzymes, but FAD is attached covalently to succinate dehydrogenase. As the coenzymes are reduced, they are effectively absorbing the potential energy which was contained in the food molecules, because the reoxidation of the coenzymes NADH and $FADH_2$ fuels the synthesis of ATP.

The reduced coenzymes transfer their electrons into the electron transfer chain (see Fig. 38.1). This is a series of proteins on the inner mitochondrial membrane organized in order of progressively increasing redox potential. NADH can reduce (and so transfer its electons to) the first complex of the chain, while $FADH_2$ can only reduce the second complex of the chain. The driving force generated by the increasing redox potentials of adjacent components of the chain carries electrons through the chain until, finally, complex IV somehow accumulates four e^- and reduces O_2, which then combines with H^+ to form H_2O. As the electons move down the redox potential gradient, energy is released and at three sites along the chain (complexes I, III and IV) the energy released is sufficient to pump H^+ across the inner mitochondrial membrane from the matrix to the intermembraneous space. The outer surface of the inner membrane subsequently becomes 140 mV more positive than the inner surface of the membrane and the intermembraneous space becomes 1.4 pH units lower than the matrix. As a result, a proton motive force of approximately 200 mV develops across the inner mitochondrial membrane. This membrane is, however, impervious to H^+ and the only way for the H^+ to cross is via a proton channel (F_0) which is coupled to ATP synthase (F_1). The ATP synthase enzyme is activated by the passage of H^+ and catalyses the phosphorylation of ADP to ATP with the passage of three protons through the channel. This method for the generation of ATP from ADP and P_i is known as **oxidative phosphorylation**. Getting ATP out of the mitochondria and ADP into the mitochondria costs one H^+, and so it takes four H^+ to produce one ATP *outside* the mitochondria. $FADH_2$ can only reduce complex II, so its reoxidation yields only two molecules of ATP while that of NADH yields about three.

Complex I is composed of a NADH dehydrogenase with a flavin mononucleotide cofactor and various Fe–S proteins. **Complex II** is composed of various FADH dehydrogenases and Fe–S proteins. **Coenzyme Q** (ubiquinone) shuttles e^- from I and II to III. **Complex III** is composed of cytochromes b and c_1. **Cytochrome c** shuttles e^- from complexes III to IV. **Complex IV** is composed of cytochromes a and a_3.

39 Glycolysis and gluconeogenesis

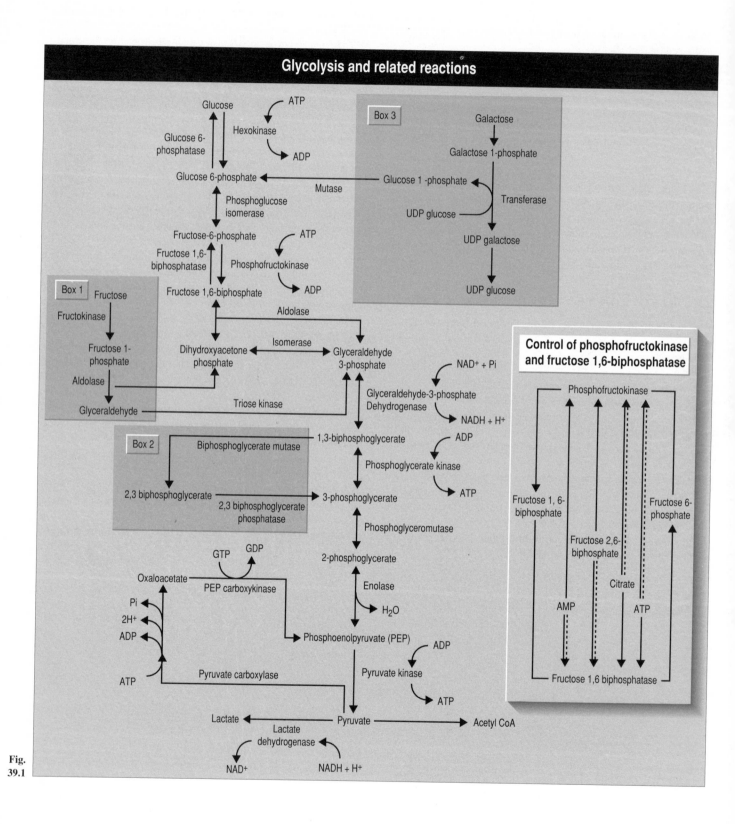

Fig.
39.1

GLYCOLYSIS

Glycolysis, which occurs in the cytosol of the cell, can be divided into two parts.

1 In the first part, the six-carbon monosaccharide is phosphorylated twice and glucopyranose is converted into fructofuranose. The addition of the phosphate groups uses two molecules of ATP. This phosphorylation prevents the sugar from leaving the cell and activates the molecule for later oxidative energy-producing reactions.

2 The initial reaction of the second part of glycolysis splits the six-carbon sugar into two triose phosphate sugars. At equilibrium, 96% of these are in the form of dihydroxyacetone phosphate. This is quickly converted into its isomer, glyceraldehyde-3-phosphate, which is oxidized to 1,3-biphosphoglycerate. As a result, the second half of the pathway is 'repeated' once for each molecule of glucose metabolized.

Substrate level phosphorylation

There are two reactions in glycolysis when ADP is phosphorylated to ATP: (i) the conversion of 1,3-bisphosphoglycerate to 3-phosphoglycerate; and (ii) the conversion of phosphoenolpyruvate to pyruvate.

The two reactions shown above phosphorylate ADP by **substrate level phosphorylation**, which is the formation of ATP by phosphate group transfer from a substrate. The first of these molecules, 1,3-biphosphoglycerate, is formed by the coupling of an endergonic reaction (the phosphorylation of a carboxylate) to an exergonic reaction (the oxidation of an aldehyde — in this case glyceraldehyde-3-phosphate). The second of the 'high-energy' molecules, phosphoenolpyruvate, generates sufficient free energy to phosphorylate ADP by its conversion to an intermediate, enolpyruvate, which can then form pyruvate. The second half of glycolysis will therefore produce four ATP, while the first half metabolizes two ATP.

In summary:

$$glucose + 2Pi + 2ADP + 2NAD^+ \rightarrow 2pyruvate + 2H_2O + 2ATP + 2NADH + 2H^+$$

There are a couple of points that should be noted about glycolysis.

1 All the reactions of glycolysis discussed above are **reversible** apart from three: those catalysed by hexokinase, by phosphofructokinase and by pyruvate kinase.

2 **No O_2 is necessary for the glycolysis to function.** This means that in tissues where O_2 is low (e.g. active muscles), poorly supplied (e.g. cornea) or where oxidative metabolism cannot occur (e.g. erythrocytes have no mitochondria), ATP can still be produced from energy sources. In anaerobic respiration, i.e. without O_2, pyruvate is reduced to lactate. This reaction oxidizes NADH, and the coenzyme can then return to the reaction catalysed by glyceraldehyde-3-phosphate dehydrogenase where it is reduced.

Integration of galactose and fructose into glycolysis

Galactose and fructose are also final products of the digestion of carbohydrates and are integrated into glycolysis (see Fig. 39.1, Boxes 1 and 3). Fructose can also be converted to fructose-6-phosphate by hexokinase, but the enzyme's affinity for fructose is much lower than for glucose.

GLUCONEOGENESIS

Under homeostatic conditions, enough carbohydrate is ingested in the diet to supply organs such as the brain, and cells such as the erythrocyte, which require glucose as their primary fuel. Under conditions of deficient dietary intake, glucose can be formed from non-carbohydrate precursors. This pathway is called gluconeogenesis and runs in the opposite direction to glycolysis (i.e. from pyruvate to glucose).

Gluconeogenesis occurs mainly in the liver, but also to a lesser extent in the kidney cortex. Some amino acids can enter this pathway through their conversion to either **oxaloacetate** or **pyruvate,** depending on their initial structure. Of the products of the digestion of triglycerides, only **glycerol** can enter gluconeogenesis through its conversion to dihydroxyacetone phosphate and subsequently to glucose. Lactate is also used in gluconeogenesis through its conversion to pyruvate.

Gluconeogenesis pathway

Although glucose is formed from pyruvate, gluconeogenesis is not simply a reversal of the reactions of glycolysis. Three of the reactions of glycolysis are irreversible and have to be bypassed or catalysed by different enzymes. They are the reactions catalysed by: (i) **hexokinase**; (ii) **phosphofructo-kinase**; and (iii) **pyruvate kinase**.

The overall change in free energy for the gluconeogenic pathway is positive and four ATP and two GTP are metabolized to fuel the pathway.

The reaction catalysed by pyruvate carboxylase occurs in the mitochondiral matrix. The other reactions in the gluconeogenic pathway occur in the cytosol. Oxaloacetate has no carrier through which it can leave the mitochondria and has to be reduced to malate by a NADH-linked dehydrogenase. Malate does have a specific carrier and leaves the mitochondria for the cytosol where it is reoxidized to oxaloacetate which can return to the gluconeogenic pathway. To convert two molecules of pyruvate to one molecule of glucose, four ATP and two GTP are needed.

REGULATORY ENZYMES OF GLYCOLYSIS AND GLUCONEOGENESIS

Glycolysis is one of the central pathways of metabolism as it provides substrates for both energy production and biosyntheses. It is therefore vital that both glycolysis and gluconeogenesis are controlled to prevent wasting of fuel molecules or excessive production of macromolecule precursors.

The main step that controls glycolysis and gluconeogenesis is shown in Fig. 39.1. ATP acts at regulatory sites via an allosteric mechanism, thereby preventing excessive energy production when the ATP/AMP ratio is high. Citrate enchances the action of ATP, thus preventing the over-formation of carbon skeletons for biosyntheses, whose levels are reflected by citrate levels. Fructose-2,6-bisphosphate acts to stimulate glycolysis when levels of fructose-6-phosphate rise.

There are two other enzymes that play a smaller part in the control of glycolysis: hexokinase and pyruvate kinase. Hexokinase is inhibited by glucose-6-phosphate, but when glucose levels rise over a critical level in the liver, the same reaction can be catalysed by glucokinase, which has a higher K_m for glucose than hexokinase. The product of the reaction catalysed by pyruvate kinase is pyruvate, which can be used to build molecules or produce energy by its conversion to acetyl CoA. Pyruvate kinase exists in three forms: L (mostly in the liver), M (in muscle) and A (in other tissues). The L form is allosterically inhibited by ATP, thus slowing the production of energy when levels of ATP are high.

40 The citric acid cycle and mitochondrial carriers

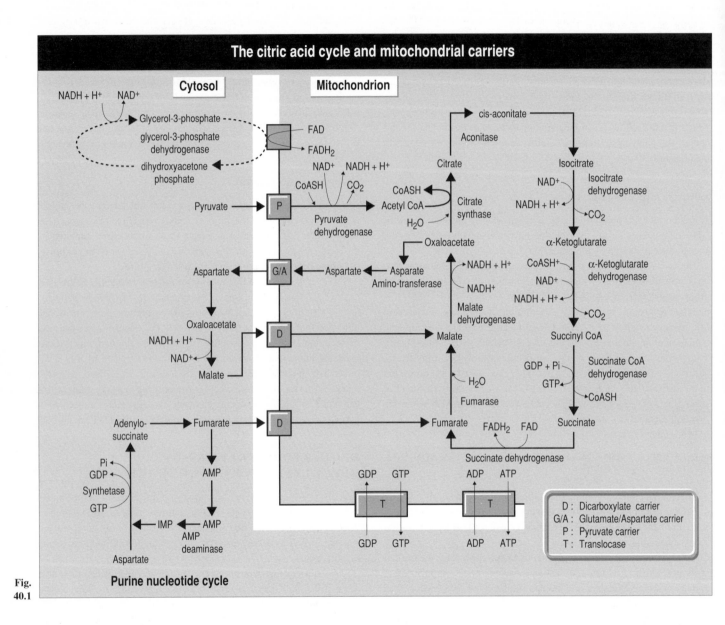

Fig. 40.1

INTRODUCTION

The citric acid cycle is a series of reactions in the matrix of the mitochondria that completes the oxidation of carbohydrates, fatty acids and amino acid skeletons, and in so doing reduces electron carriers so that they can fuel the redox chain. Pyruvate in the cytosol is shuttled into the matrix of the mitochondria where it is converted into acetyl CoA. Acetyl CoA then enters the citric acid cycle by condensing with oxaloacetate to form citrate. The subsequent reactions of the cycle are a series of modifications to the carbon skeleton, which results in the regeneration of oxaloacetate. The overall reaction achieved by one round of the citric acid cycle is:

$$3NAD^+ + FAD + acetyl\ CoA + GDP + 2H_2O + Pi \rightarrow$$
$$3NADH + 2CO_2 + FADH_2 + CoA + GTP + 2H^+$$

Products and stoichiometry

There are a number of important points that need to be noted about the products and stoichiometry of the citric acid cycle.

1 Within one cycle there are four dehydrogenation reactions, which result in the reduction of three NAD^+ and one FAD. These hydrogen carriers exist in only limited quantities in the mitochondria and need to be reoxidized in the eletron transport chain for the citric acid cycle to continue. Consequently, the **citric acid cycle can only operate under aerobic conditions.**

2 Two carbon atoms in the form of acetyl CoA enter the cycle and two different carbon atoms leave the cycle in the form of CO_2. The decarboxylation reactions are those which are catalysed by α-ketoglutarate dehydrogenase and by isocitrate dehydrogenase.

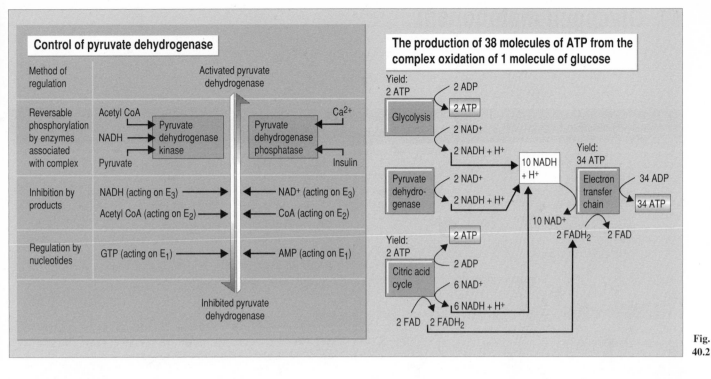

Control of pyruvate dehydrogenase

Method of regulation	Activated pyruvate dehydrogenase		
Reversable phosphorylation by enzymes associated with complex	Acetyl CoA, NADH, Pyruvate → Pyruvate dehydrogenase kinase	Pyruvate dehydrogenase phosphatase	← Ca²⁺, ← Insulin
Inhibition by products	NADH (acting on E₃) →	← NAD⁺ (acting on E₃)	
	Acetyl CoA (acting on E₂) →	← CoA (acting on E₂)	
Regulation by nucleotides	GTP (acting on E₁) →	← AMP (acting on E₁)	

Inhibited pyruvate dehydrogenase

The production of 38 molecules of ATP from the complex oxidation of 1 molecule of glucose

Yield: 2 ATP — Glycolysis → 2 ADP → 2 ATP; 2 NAD⁺ → 2 NADH + H⁺

Pyruvate dehydrogenase: 2 NAD⁺ → 2 NADH + H⁺ → 10 NADH + H⁺

Yield: 34 ATP — Electron transfer chain → 34 ADP → 34 ATP; 10 NAD⁺; 2 FADH₂ → 2 FAD

Yield: 2 ATP — Citric acid cycle → 2 ATP; 2 ADP; 6 NAD⁺ → 6 NADH + H⁺; 2 FAD, 2 FADH₂

Fig. 40.2

3 The two reactions catalysed by citrate synthase and by fumarase each consume one molecule of H_2O.

4 A molecule of GTP is formed from a molecule of GDP and Pi in the reaction catalysed by succinyl CoA synthetase.

ENZYMES OF THE CITRIC ACID CYCLE AND THEIR CONTROL

The citric acid cycle is vital in the process of **energy generation**, but is also intricately involved in other fundamental metabolic processes such as **gluconeogenesis**, **amino acid metabolism** and **lipogenesis**. It is therefore important that the cycle be precisely controlled so as not to provide an excess of biosynthetic precursors nor to utilize more fuel than is absolutely necessary. There are four main enzymes by which the cycle is controlled: (i) the pyruvate dehydrogenase complex; (ii) citrate synthase; (iii) isocitrate dehydrogenase; and (iv) α-ketoglutarate dehydrogenase.

1 The irreversible conversion of pyruvate to acetyl CoA by the pyruvate dehydrogenase complex is not part of the citric acid cycle but is essential for its efficient functioning. The complex is made up of three enzymes:

(a) E_1 — pyruvate dehydrogenase oxidatively decarboxylates pyruvate;

(b) E_2 — dihydrolipoyl transacetylase transfers the acetyl residue to acetyl CoA; and

(c) E_3 — dihydrolipoyl dehydrogenase oxidatively regenerates a lipoamide.

2 Citrate synthase controls the entry of acetyl CoA into the cycle, and is inhibited allosterically by ATP.

3 Isocitrate dehydrogenase catalyses the conversion of isocitrate to α-ketoglutarate. The enzyme is allosterically stimulated by ADP and is competitively inhibited by NADH which can displace NAD⁺.

4 α-Ketoglutarate dehydrogenase catalyses the conversion of α-ketoglutarate to succinyl CoA. It exists as a three-enzyme complex similar to pyruvate dehydrogenase, and shares many of its properties, i.e. its activity is regulated by its products and also by levels of phosphorylated nucleotides in the cell.

THE GLYCEROL-3-PHOSPHATE SHUNT AND THE MALATE/ASPARTATE SHUNT

The glycolytic reaction that oxidizes glyceraldehyde-3-phosphate to 1,3-biphosphoglycerate results in the reduction of NAD⁺ to NADH. Quantities of this hydrogen carrier are limited in the cytosol and therefore NADH needs to be reoxidized for glycolysis to be maintained.

The oxidation of NADH in the electron chain occurs in the mitochondria, but the carrier cannot pass across the inner mitochondrial membrane. Thus, two systems have developed so that the cytosolic NADH can be reoxidized in the mitochondria.

1 In the **glycerol-3-phosphate shunt**, a cytosolic dehydrogenase oxidizes NADH as dihydroxyacetone phosphate is reduced to glycerol-3-phosphate. A mitochondrial dehydrogenase operates in the reverse direction, but reduces FAD instead of NAD⁺.

2 In the **malate/aspartate shunt** NADH is oxidized by the conversion of oxaloacetate to malate. Malate crosses the inner mitochondrial membrane where it is oxidized to oxaloacetate. Oxaloacetate is then transaminated to form aspartate, which moves back into the cytosol.

PURINE NUCLEOTIDE CYCLE

The purine nucleotide cycle is used to supply fumarate to the citric acid cycle when the availability of acetyl CoA exceeds the availability of oxaloacetate. This imbalance commonly occurs in skeletal muscle during exercise, and the nucleotide cycle is essential for maintaining the efficient functioning of the citric acid cycle.

41 Glycogen metabolism

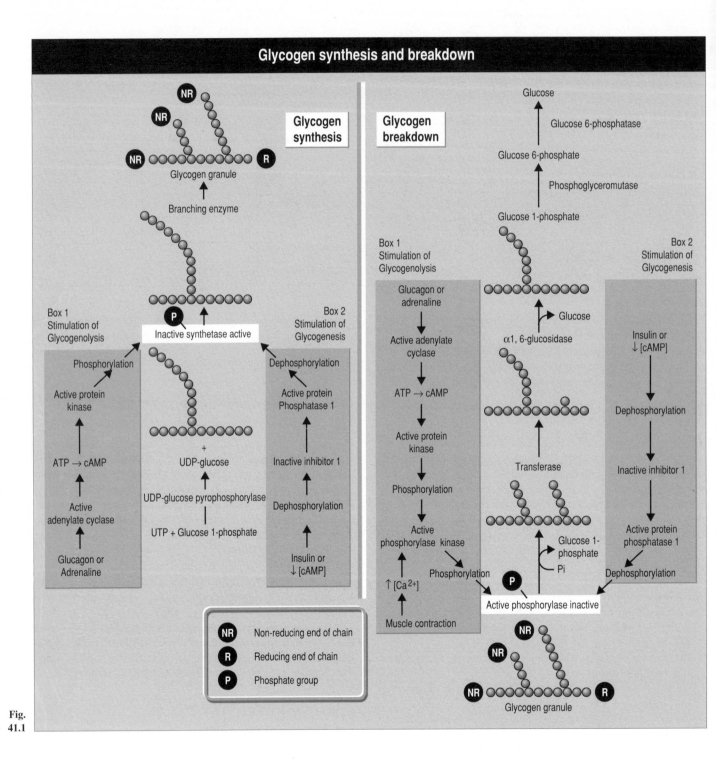

Fig. 41.1

INTRODUCTION

Glycogen is the form in which glucose is stored. It is composed of many glucose residues joined by α-1,4-glycosidic bonds (see Chapter 36) with α-1,6-linked branch points. Glycogen exists in the cytosol of the cell as granules. These granules range from 10 to 40 nm in size and contain the enzymes that are involved in glycogen metabolism. The main sources of glycogen in the body are the liver (100 g after a meal) and skeletal muscle (up to 300 g), although there are also substantial amounts in cells of the intestines, kidneys and brain.

GLYCOGENOLYSIS

1 Phosphorylase catalyses the removal of a glucose residue by the phosphorylysis of an α-1,4-glycosidic bond. Phosphorylase requires the presence of the coenzyme pyridoxal phosphate, which acts as an acid–base catalyst, to work.

2 Phosphorylase can only break α-1,4-glycosidic bonds up to four residues away from a branch point. The three residues leading to the branch are then transferred to another part of the glycogen molecule by transferase.

3 The α-1,6-glycosidic bond forming the branch point is cleaved by α-1,6-glucosidase.

4 Phosphoglucomutase converts glucose-1-phosphate into glucose-6-phosphate, via a glucose-1,6-biphosphate intermediate, which can then enter glycolysis. In the liver, intestines and kidney, glucose-6-phosphatase can remove a phosphate group from glucose-6-phosphate to form glucose, which can then pass out of the cell into the bloodstream. In brain and skeletal muscle tissue, glucose-6-phosphatase is not present and glucose-6-phosphate cannot pass out of the cells.

GLYCOGEN SYNTHESIS

The synthesis of glycogen (glycogenesis) follows a different pathway from that of glycogenolysis.

1 To be added onto a chain in a glycogen molecule, the glucose residue must be in the 'activated' form of uridine diphosphate (UDP)–glucose.

glucose-1-phosphate + UTP → UDP–glucose + pyrophosphate

This is catalysed by UDP–glucose pyrophosphorylase. The reaction is driven towards the formation of UDP–glucose by the hydrolysis of pyrophosphate to orthophosphate by the enzyme pyrophosphatase.

2 Glycogen synthase catalyses the addition of glucose from UDP–glucose to the non-reducing end of a chain. The α-1,4-glycosidic bond is made with the hydroxyl group on C_4 and UDP is released. Glycogen synthase can only add UDP–glucose to a chain of five or more residues. Chains smaller than five residues are attached to proteins and are called primers.

3 When a chain contains more than 11 residues, a branching enzyme transfers a block of seven to an interior site within the glycogen molecule, to form a new branch. The branch point must be at least four residues away from any pre-existing branch points.

CONTROL OF GLYCOGEN METABOLISM

The synthesis and breakdown of glycogen is one of the major controlling factors that determine the availability of glucose for energy production in the body. When there is an excess of carbohydrates in the body, for example after a meal, it is important that glucose can be stored for later use. In periods such as these, **insulin** is secreted by the endocrine glands of the pancreas and causes glycogenesis.

On the other hand, if a supply of glucose is needed which is not readily available from the diet, glycogen can be broken down to give **glucose-6-phosphate**, which can be integrated directly into glycolysis or glucose, which can pass into the circulation and be taken up by organs that need it. When concentrations of glucose are low in the blood, **glucagon** is secreted from the endocrine cells of the pancreas, and in periods of stress or excitement **adrenaline** is secreted from the adrenal glands. Both glucagon and adrenaline stimulate glycogenolysis (Note: there are no glucagon receptors in muscle tissue.)

Both glucagon and adrenaline work via a **cascade mechanism** whereby the initial signal by the hormone is amplified manyfold while being relayed to the enzymes of glycogen metabolism. The hormonal signals are dually effective because reversible phosphorylation is used to control the activity of the enzymes. So, for example, when glucose is needed, the enzymes catalysing glycogenolysis are phosphorylated and activated while the enzymes catalysing glycogenesis are phosphorylated and inactivated.

Control of enzyme activity by phosphorylation

The enzyme phosphorylase in skeletal muscle can exist in two forms depending on the phosphorylation of a specific serine residue: **phosphorylase a** and **phosphorylase b**. Phosphorylase a is phosphorylated and is usually always active while phosphorylase b is dephosphorylated and is usually inactive. The two forms are interconvertible by the actions of phosphorylase kinase and phosphatase 1, which also control the activity of glycogen synthase. In turn, the activity of phosphorylase kinase and phosphatase 1 are also controlled by reversible phosphorylation. The activity of phosphatase 1 is modulated by a protein called inhibitor 1. When inhibitor 1 is phosphorylated (e.g. by the action of cAMP-activated protein kinase) it inhibits the activity of phosphatase 1. However, when levels of cAMP fall, or when insulin acts on the cell, inhibitor 1 becomes dephosphorylated and the phosphatase 1 activity resumes. When glucose levels are high, the activity of phosphorylase falls before the activity of synthase rises. This is explained below.

1 Glucose enters the cell and binds to the phosphorylase component of a phosphorylase a: phosphatase 1 complex.

2 Phosphatase 1 dephosphorylates phosphorylase a to yield inactive phosphorylase b.

3 Phosphorylase b dissociates from phosphatase 1.

4 Phosphatase 1 then dephosphorylates glycogen synthase b to convert it into the active glycogen synthase a form.

PATHOPHYSIOLOGY

Von Gierke's disease is a deficiency of the glucose-6-phosphatase enzyme in liver and kidney tissues. The resulting increased levels of glycogen in the affected organs causes enlargement of the organs and hypoglycaemia. **Cori's disease** is a deficiency of the debranching enzyme in liver and muscle tissues. Increased levels of glycogen with short branches result and cause similar symptoms to type 1 disease. **McArdle's disease** is a deficiency in muscle phosphorylase. Only moderately increased levels of glycogen result in the muscle tissue, but severe cramps develop with exercise due to the lack of glucose-6-phosphate available for oxidation.

42 Lipid metabolism I

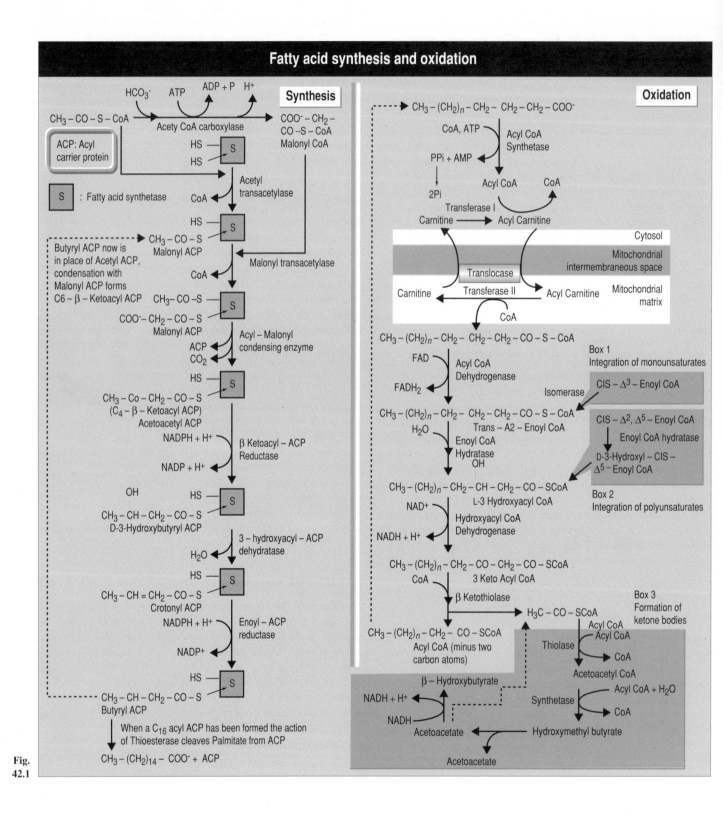

Fatty acid synthesis and oxidation

Fig. 42.1

BREAKDOWN OF LIPIDS

Formation of fatty acids and glycerol from triglycerides

The breakdown of lipids begins with the hydrolysis of a cytosolic triglyceride into one molecule of glycerol and three fatty acids. This reaction is catalysed by the enzyme **hormone-sensitive lipase**, which is activated by **glucagon**, **adrenaline**, **noradrenaline** and **adrenocorticotrophin (ACTH)**. These hormones and neurotransmitters act via a cAMP cascade mechanism which leads to the phosphorylation of the enzyme. **Insulin** action results in the dephosphorylation and inactivation of the enzyme.

Glycerol can enter glycolysis by phosphorylation to glycerol-3-phosphate. This is then oxidized to form dihydroxyacetone phosphate.

Fatty acid oxidation

The fatty acids are 'activated' by the formation of a thioester bond between the carboxyl group of the acid to the sulphydryl group of CoA. The reaction is catalysed by acyl CoA synthetase and is driven forward by the hydrolysis of pyrophosphate. The subsequent shuttling of the fatty acid into the mitochondrial matrix and its breakdown (called ß-oxidation) are shown in Fig. 42.1. Carnitine deficiency or a defect in the translocase enzyme impairs energy production from fat oxidation and results in muscle cramps developing with exercise. The overall reaction for the oxidation of a typical fatty acid is shown below:

$$\text{palmitoyl CoA} + 7NAD^+ + 7FAD + 7H_2O + 7CoA \rightarrow$$
$$8\text{acetyl CoA} + 7NADH + 7H^+ + 7FADH_2$$

The complete oxidation of this fatty acid will thus yield 129 molecules of ATP.

Many fatty acids occur that contain one or more double bonds in the hydrocarbon tail and are said to be **unsaturated**. The enzymes of the ß-oxidation chain are stereospecific and the unsaturated fatty acids have to be modified before they can be fully oxidized. The modification of an acid with only one double bond is shown in Fig. 42.1, Box 1, while those of polyunsaturates are shown in Fig. 42.1, Box 2.

The rate of breakdown is determined by the availability of substrates, the inhibition of carnitine transferase 1 by malonyl CoA and the inhibition of hydroxyacyl CoA dehydrogenase by NADH.

Ketone body formation

When the breakdown of fats exceeds the breakdown of carbohydrates, the supply of acetyl CoA from β-oxidation exceeds the rate that oxaloacetate can be formed. The acetyl CoA then follows a different pathway; that of ketone body formation (Fig. 42.1, Box 3). The ketone bodies, acetoacetate and hydroxybutyrate, diffuse out of the cell and are common fuel molecules in the body, especially in cardiac muscle and the renal cortex where acetyl CoA can be regenerated. The regeneration of acetyl CoA from acetoacetate is catalysed by two enzymes: (i) CoA transferase adds a CoA group; and (ii) thiolase cleaves acetoacetyl CoA, incorporating another CoA, to form two molecules of acetyl CoA.

THE SYNTHESIS OF FATTY ACIDS

There are three major differences between fatty acid synthesis and breakdown:

1 synthesis occurs in the cytosol whereas breakdown occurs in the mitochondria;

2 the enzymes catalysing the breakdown are separate whereas those catalysing the synthesis are joined to form a single polypeptide chain called fatty acid synthase;

3 the reductant used in the synthesis is NADPH whereas the electron donors in the breakdown are FAD and NAD^+.

The principal reactions of fatty acid synthesis are shown in Fig. 42.1 Essentially, the pathway consists of the repetitive addition of a two-carbon unit to the forming fatty acid by the condensation of a three-carbon unit (malonyl CoA) to the end of the fatty acid tail and the release of CO_2.

The committed step of the pathway is the irreversible conversion of acetyl CoA to malonyl CoA. The enzyme catalysing this reaction, acetyl CoA carboxylase, has a prosthetic biotin group attached, which is initially carboxylated by a biotin carboxylase subunit of the enzyme. A transcarboxylase subunit of the enzyme then transfers the CO_2 group to the acetyl CoA.

After the formation of malonyl CoA, the next step in the synthesis pathway is the activation of the substrates by their attachment to the phosphopantetheine group of acyl carrier protein (ACP). The subsequent steps are shown in Fig. 42.1 and the overall reaction for the synthesis of palmitate is as follows:

$$8\text{acetyl CoA} + 14NADPH + 7ATP \rightarrow \text{palmitate} + 8CoA + 6H_2O$$
$$+ 14NADP^+ + 7ADP + Pi$$

Fatty acid synthase

This enzyme is dimeric with each subunit composed of three domains.
1 **Domain 1**: acetyl CoA transferase, malonyl CoA transferase, acylmalonyl condensing enzyme.
2 **Domain 2**: ACP, β-ketoacyl reductase, hydroxyacyl dehydratase, enoyl reductase.
3 **Domain 3**: thioesterase.

The dimer is arranged so that the domain 1 of one of the enzymes is facing domains 2 and 3 of the other enzyme. Therefore, by rotating on the phosphopantetheinyl group, the activating reactions can occur on one of the enzymes and the rest of the reactions in the cycle can occur on the opposite enzyme.

The main site of control in fatty acid synthesis is the enzyme acetyl CoA carboxylase. The enzyme's activity is inhibited by high levels of palmitoyl CoA and the actions of glucagon, and is stimulated by high levels of citrate and the actions of insulin.

The assembly of triglycerides: the α-glycerol phosphate pathway

Triglycerides are formed by the esterification of three fatty acyl CoA molecules with one molecule of α-glycerol phosphate.
1 α-Glycerol phosphate can be formed by the phosphorylation of glycerol or by the dehydrogenation of dihydroxy acetone phosphate by NADH.
2 α-Glycerol phosphate combines with two molecules of fatty acyl CoA to form **phosphatidate** and two molecules of CoA.
3 The phosphate group is removed to form a **diglyceride**.
4 The diglyceride combines with a third molecule of fatty acyl CoA to form a **triglyceride** and a molecule of CoA.

43 Lipid metabolism II

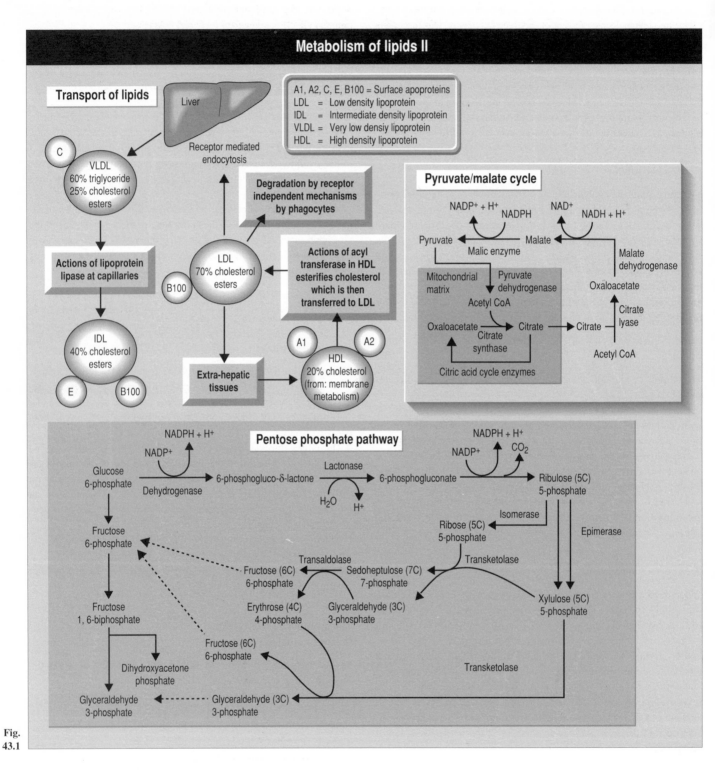

Metabolism of lipids II

Transport of lipids

Liver

A1, A2, C, E, B100 = Surface apoproteins
LDL = Low density lipoprotein
IDL = Intermediate density lipoprotein
VLDL = Very low densiy lipoprotein
HDL = High density lipoprotein

C

VLDL
60% triglyceride
25% cholesterol
esters

Receptor mediated
endocytosis

Degradation by receptor
independent mechanisms
by phagocytes

Pyruvate/malate cycle

$NADP^+ + H^+$ NADPH NAD^+ $NADH + H^+$

Pyruvate   Malate
Malic enzyme

Actions of lipoprotein
lipase at capillaries

LDL
70% cholesterol
esters

B100

Actions of acyl
transferase in HDL
esterifies cholesterol
which is then
transferred to LDL

Malate
dehydrogenase

Oxaloacetate

Mitochondrial   Pyruvate
matrix   dehydrogenase
            Acetyl CoA

Citrate
lyase

IDL
40% cholesterol
esters

Oxaloacetate   Citrate   Citrate

A1   A2

Citrate
synthase

Acetyl CoA

E   B100

Extra-hepatic
tissues

HDL
20% cholesterol
(from: membrane
metabolism)

Citric acid cycle enzymes

Pentose phosphate pathway

$NADPH + H^+$

$NADP^+$

Glucose
6-phosphate

Lactonase

6-phosphogluco-δ-lactone

$NADPH + H^+$

$NADP^+$ CO_2

6-phosphogluconate

Ribulose (5C)
5-phosphate

Dehydrogenase

H_2O H^+

Isomerase

Ribose (5C)
5-phosphate

Epimerase

Fructose
6-phosphate

Transaldolase

Fructose (6C)
6-phosphate

Sedoheptulose (7C)
7-phosphate

Transketolase

Fructose
1, 6-biphosphate

Erythrose (4C)
4-phosphate

Glyceraldehyde (3C)
3-phosphate

Xylulose (5C)
5-phosphate

Fructose (6C)
6-phosphate

Dihydroxyacetone
phosphate

Transketolase

Glyceraldehyde
3-phosphate

Glyceraldehyde (3C)
3-phosphate

**Fig.
43.1**

In this chapter, two principles are discussed: (i) the formation of reducing power for biosyntheses in the form of NADPH; and (ii) the carriage of lipids around the body.

PRODUCTION OF NADPH FROM NADP⁺

NADPH differs from NADH only in that there is a phosphate group attached to C_2, but their uses in metabolism are clearly differentiated. Both molecules can provide reducing power to fuel reactions by their oxidation to $NADP^+$ and NAD^+, but the reducing power from the oxidation of NADPH is used to fuel biosyntheses while that from NADH is used to fuel the reactions involved in the generation of ATP.

There are two different metabolic pathways that reduce $NADP^+$ to NADPH: (i) the pyruvate malate cycle; and (ii) the pentose phosphate pathway. Approximately 40% of the NADPH needed for fatty acid synthesis is produced by the pyruvate malate cycle (see Fig. 43.1). The remainder is produced by the pentose phosphate pathway.

The pentose phosphate pathway

The pentose phosphate pathway is made up of two component pathways: (i) an oxidative pathway; and (ii) a non-oxidative pathway. These both occur in the cytosol. The oxidative pathway is responsible for the formation of NADPH and involves the irreversible conversion of **glucose-6-phosphate**, through a series of steps, to **ribulose-5-phosphate**. Ribulose-5-phosphate is a precursor for a number of important molecules in the body, which include DNA, RNA, ATP and CoA. If synthesis of these molecules is required in the cell, then ribulose-5-phosphate will be utilized for that purpose. If ribulose-5-phosphate is not required for biosyntheses, the **non-oxidative pathway** is used.

The non-oxidative pathway is a series of reversible carbon skeleton interconversions which result in the formation of two molecules of fructose-6-phosphate and one molecule of glyceraldehyde-3-phosphate from three molecules of ribulose-5-phosphate. The starting substrate of the oxidative pathway and the products of the non-oxidative pathway are all metabolites of the glycolytic pathway, and so the pentose phosphate pathway can act as a shunt off from glycolysis.

The rate-limiting step for the oxidative pathway is the conversion of glucose-6-phosphate to 6-phosphoglucolactone. This reaction is catalysed by the enzyme glucose-6-phosphate dehydrogenase, whose activity is regulated by levels of $NADP^+$. The controlling factors in the non-oxidative pathway are the availabilities of the substrates.

Pathophysiology of the pentose phosphate pathway. A deficiency of the enzyme glucose-6-phosphate dehydrogenase in red blood cells is found in 11% of black Americans. This deficiency leads to decreased levels of NADPH in the red blood cells. NADPH is needed in these cells for the reduction of oxidized glutathione. Glutathione maintains the reduced state of the cell and is also involved in the metabolism of toxins. The deficiency therefore predisposes the cell to damage which might be prevented with sufficient levels of reduced glutathione.

Wernicke–Korsakoff syndrome. The enzyme ketolase, of the non-oxidative pathway, tightly binds a thiamine pyrophosphate prosthetic group. In the Wernicke–Korsakoff syndrome, the prosthetic group is held less tightly than normal and a deficiency of thiamine in the diet (e.g. in alcoholics or malnourishment) precipitates characteristic symptoms which include disorientation and decreased mental function.

CARRIAGE OF LIPIDS AROUND THE BODY

Lipids are transported round the body in structures known as **lipoproteins**. These lipoproteins consist of a **shell** of polar lipids (phospholipids and free cholesterol) and apoproteins and a **core** of non-polar lipids (triglycerides and cholesterol esters). Carriage of the lipids in this way facilitates their transport in an aqueous medium and enables a very specific targeting system for metabolites to occur. Dietary lipids that have been digested and absorbed follow an exogenous pathway involving chylomicrons and chylomicron remnants.

Lipids that have been formed within the body, for example biosynthesis in the liver or membrane turnover, follow an endogenous pathway. This pathway involves four different types of lipoprotein which can be differentiated by density and surface protein markers: (i) very low-density lipoprotein (VLDL); (ii) intermediate-density lipoprotein (IDL); (iii) low-density lipoprotein (LDL); (iv) high-density lipoprotein (HDL).

The passage and interconversions of the lipoproteins are shown in Fig. 43.1. As triglycerides are lost from the core of the lipoproteins, VLDL become IDL, which lose more triglyceride to become LDL. Nascent HDL is released in the liver and acquires further lipid from the mebranes of peripheral cells; its purpose is to transfer cholesterol esters to other lipoproteins for subsequent hepatic metabolism.

Pathophysiology of lipid transport

Familial hypercholesterolaemia (type IIa) is caused by a deficiency of the LDL receptor as a result of a number of types of mutation (e.g. absent receptor; defective ligand binding by receptor; disruption of transport to cell membrane of receptor). Increased blood levels of LDL and cholesterol result and these may be deposited in the walls of arteries leading to premature atheroma.

Familial hyperlipoproteinaemia (type III) is caused by an abnormal apoprotein E and causes increased blood levels of remnant particles (IDL) with raised triglycerides and cholesterol levels.

Familial hypertriglyceridaemia (type IV) has an unknown cause, but results in increased blood levels of VLDL with high triglycerides.

44 Nucleotide synthesis

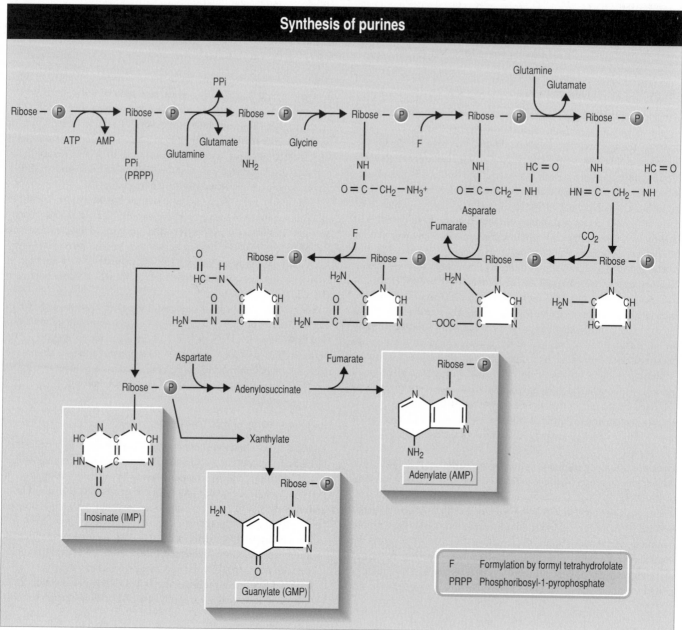

Fig. 44.1

Nucleotides are involved in most of the integral biochemical processes of the cell. To name only a few of their functions, they are involved in energy storage and release (ATP), communication of extracellular signals intracellulary (cAMP) and genetic information processing (DNA and RNA). The structure of nucleotides is described in Chapter 6.

ASSEMBLY OF PURINES

The purine ring is assembled from five precursors: glycine, glutamine, aspartate, CO_2 and formyltetrahydrofolate. The first step in the synthesis is the formation of **5-phosphoribosyl-1-pyrophosphate (PRPP)** from **ribose-5-phosphate** and is catalysed by the enzyme **ribose phosphate pyrophosphokinase.**

The second step is the committed step in the synthesis and is the irreversible formation of **5-phosphoribosylamine** from PRPP. This

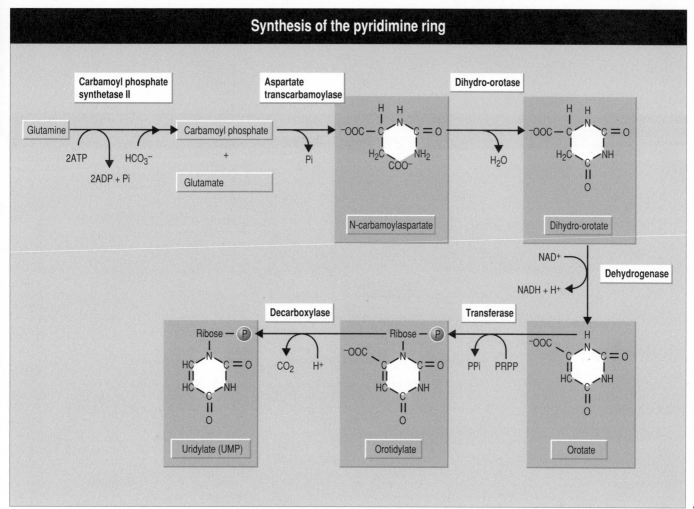

Synthesis of the pyridimine ring

Fig. 44.2

reaction is catalysed by **amidophosphoribosyl transferase** and is driven forward by pyrophosphate hydrolysis.

Control of purine ring synthesis

The synthesis of the purine ring is controlled mainly at four sites:

1 ribose phosphate pyrophosphokinase is inhibited by AMP, inosine monophosphate (IMP) and GMP;

2 amidophosphoribosyl transferase is inhibited by AMP, IMP and GMP;

3 the enzyme converting IMP to adenylosuccinate is inhibited by AMP; and

4 the enzyme converting IMP to xanthylate is inhibited by IMP.

Salvage reactions

A common feature of purine nucleotide synthesis is **salvage reactions.** The breakdown of nucleotides forms free purine bases, and these can be salvaged by their direct addition to PRPP. The enzymes catalysing these reactions are adenine phosphoribosyl transferase (which forms

AMP) and hypoxanthine–guanine phosphoribosyl transferase (HGPRTase) (which forms IMP and GMP).

ASSEMBLY OF PYRIMIDINES

The synthesis of pyrimidines differs from the synthesis of purines in that the pyrimidine ring is synthesized first and is then attached to ribose phosphate. The three enzymes that catalyse the conversion of glutamine to dihydroorotate (synthetase, transcarbamoylase and dihydroorotase) are domains on one protein. The two enzymes that catalyse the conversion of orotate to uridine monophosphate (UMP) (transferase and decarboxylase) are domains on another protein.

The committed step in this synthetic pathway is the formation of carbamoylaspartate from aspartate and carbamoyl phosphate.

Note: the term 'committed step' means the first irreversible step of the pathway, and is often the step at which the pathway is controlled.

The enzyme that catalyses this reaction, aspartate transcarbamoylase, is inhibited by cytidine triphosphate (CTP). CTP is formed from UTP and is one of the end products of pyrimidine nucleotide synthesis.

45 Breakdown of nucleotides

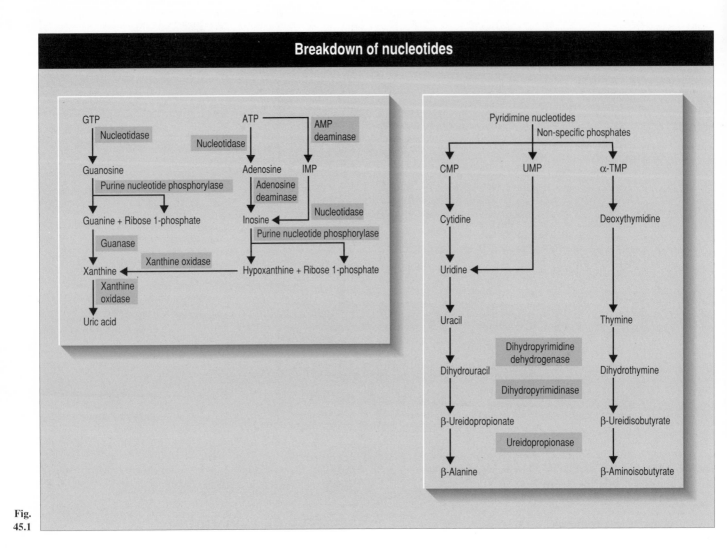

Breakdown of nucleotides

Fig.
45.1

The end product for the degradation of purines is uric acid which is excreted in the urine. The end products of degradation of pyrimidines are amino acids. The enzyme deoxyuridine triphosphatase (dUTPase) catalyses the reaction that converts dUTP to dUMP. It is important that deoxyuridine diphosphate (dUDP) is not present in the cell in high concentrations otherwise it would become incorporated into DNA. The three enzymes that catalyse the final reactions of pyrimidine breakdown (dihydropyrimidine dehydrogenase, dihydropyrimidinase and ureidopropionase) can metabolize uracil or thymine and their proceeding intermediates equally.

PATHOPHYSIOLOGY

Deficiency of adenosine deaminase

The deficiency of this enzyme results in immune impairment. It is thought that this is a result of substrate accumulation which subsequently inhibits other enzymes involved in nucleotide synthesis. Similar to this is a deficiency of purine nucleotide phosphorylase which also results in immune impairment.

Gout

Gout results from deposition of uric acid crystals in joints (causing severe pain and inflammation) as a result of increased levels of uric acid in the blood. It is often due to a metabolic abnormality which has resulted in an increased production of purine nucleotides. The uric acid may precipitate to form sodium urate crystals which are deposited in joints and kidneys and cause pain and renal impairment.

The biochemical basis for the majority of cases of primary gout is unknown, but the condition is associated with increased uric acid production and/or reduced renal excretion. In rare instances, primary gout may result from specific enzyme defects.

1 A PRPP synthase enzyme which is insensitive to feedback inhibition by GDP or ADP.

2 A partial deficiency of HGPRTase. The decreased rate of the salvage reaction causes increased levels of PRPP which will result in an increase in the activity of PRPP aminotransferase.

The symptoms of gout can be relieved by the drug allopurinol. This is metabolized by xanthine oxidase to alloxanthine which does' not dissociate from the active site of the enzyme.

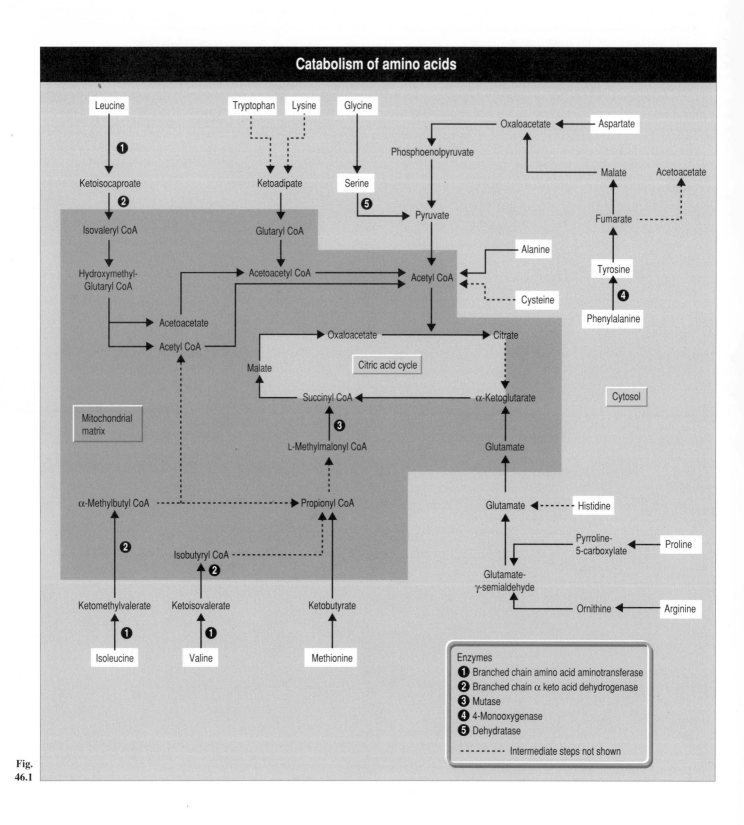

Fig. 46.1

INTRODUCTION

Amino acids in the body that are not used in protein synthesis are not stored or excreted. Instead, they are metabolized to intermediates which can be fully oxidized to provide energy or are converted to glucose, fatty acids or ketone bodies. This occurs mainly in the liver.

The pathway for the breakdown of most amino acids can be divided into two distinct phases: (i) the removal of the amino group and its conversion into urea (the Krebs–Henseleit urea cycle); and (ii) the conversion of the remaining carbon skeleton into pyruvate, one of the metabolites of the citric acid cycle, acetyl CoA or acetoacetyl CoA.

REMOVAL OF AMINO GROUP AND FORMATION OF UREA

Deamination of amino acids

The removal of the α-amino group from most amino acids is achieved by a **transamination reaction**. This reaction is catalysed by specific aminotransferases and involves transferring the amino group onto α-ketoglutarate to form **glutamate**. The loss of the amino group converts the amino acid into an α-keto-acid. The transamination catalysed by alanine aminotransferase is shown below:

alanine + α-ketoglutarate → pyruvate + glutamate

The aminotransferases are dependent on a pyridoxal phosphate prosthetic group which is derived from vitamin B_6 and can accept the amino group and transfer it to α-ketoglutarate. The amino acids serine and threonine are exceptions to the rule in that their amino groups can be converted directly to NH_4^+ by **dehydratases**.

Starvation: role of muscle aminotransferases

The importance of the aminotransferases can be seen when the body is subjected to a period of starvation. After the glycogen reserves have been depleted it is vital to maintain an adequate concentration of glucose in the blood. The body is not able to convert fatty acids to glucose, so gluconeogenesis must be fuelled by amino acids. The sequence of metabolic events is outlined below.

1 Amino acids of the muscle tissue, especially the branched chain amino acids (valine, leucine and isoleucine), are deaminated.
2 The carbon skeletons of the deaminated amino acids are metabolized by the enzymes of the citric acid cycle, phosphoenolpyruvate carboxykinase and pyruvate kinase to form pyruvate.
3 In a reaction catalysed by alanine aminotransferase, pyruvate can be converted to alanine.
4 Alanine is then released into the blood where it passes to the liver. There it is converted back to pyruvate which can then be metabolized to glucose.

The Krebs–Henseleit urea cycle

The glutamate formed by the transamination reactions can either be converted to glutamine or to α-ketoglutarate. The conversion to glutamine is fuelled by the hydrolysis of a high-energy bond of ATP and is catalysed by glutamine synthetase. Glutamine can then be used as a fuel source in the intestines or as a regulator of acid–base balance in the kidney. The conversion of glutamate to α-ketoglutarate is catalysed

by glutamate dehydrogenase, and the NH_4^+ which is formed enters the urea cycle. The formation of oxaloacetate from fumarate provides the urea cycle with a link to the citric acid cycle as oxaloacetate can condense with acetyl CoA to form citrate.

The rate at which the urea cycle functions is controlled by acetyl glutamate which stimulates carbamoyl phosphate synthetase. Acetyl glutamate is synthesized from glutamate in a reaction catalysed by a synthetase enzyme. The activity of this enzyme is increased by amino acids, particularly arginine.

INTEGRATION OF THE KETO-ACID SKELETONS INTO METABOLISM

All of the amino acids found in the body are broken down into one or more of seven intermediates in metabolism. They are acetyl CoA, acetoacetyl CoA, pyruvate, α-ketoglutarate, succinyl CoA, fumarate and oxaloacetate.

The amino acids that are degraded purely to either acetyl CoA or acetoacetyl CoA are termed **ketogenic** since their breakdown is directed towards the formation of ketone bodies. Amino acids whose breakdown products can be directed towards the formation of glucose are termed **glucogenic**. The only purely ketogenic amino acids are leucine and lysine, although isoleucine, tryptophan, phenylalanine and tyrosine are ketogenic and glucogenic.

PATHOPHYSIOLOGY

Deficiencies of the urea cycle

Any deficiency of the urea cycle is detrimental to the body, since high concentrations of NH_4^+ are toxic and the urea cycle is the only metabolic pathway which can convert NH_4^+ to a substance that can be excreted. A total deficiency of one of the enzymes of the cycle results in death shortly after birth. Partial deficiencies result in mental retardation and frequent vomiting.

Maple syrup disease

In maple syrup disease, there is a deficiency of the branched chain **α-keto-acid dehydrogenase enzyme**. This leads to an increase in the levels of isoleucine, leucine, valine and their α-keto-acid derivatives in both the blood and urine. The accumulation of these compounds in the urine causes the urine to smell similar to maple syrup, hence the name. If undetected, maple syrup disease leads to physical and mental retardation. This disease can be detected by adding 2,4-dinitrophenylhydrazine to a urine sample. This compound will combine with α-ketoisocaproate, a derivative of leucine, forming 2,4-dinitrophenylhydrazine. Management of maple syrup disease involves a specially formulated diet which is low in leucine, valine and isoleucine.

Phenylketonuria

Phenylketonuria is caused by a deficiency of the **phenylalanine mono-oxygenase enzyme**, or less commonly of its tetrahydrobiopterin cofactor. The disease has an incidence of around 1 in 25 000 newborn babies and shows an autosomal recessive inheritance pattern. In the healthy state, 75% of phenylalanine is converted into tyrosine which can then be metabolized, and the remainder of the phenylalanine is incorporated

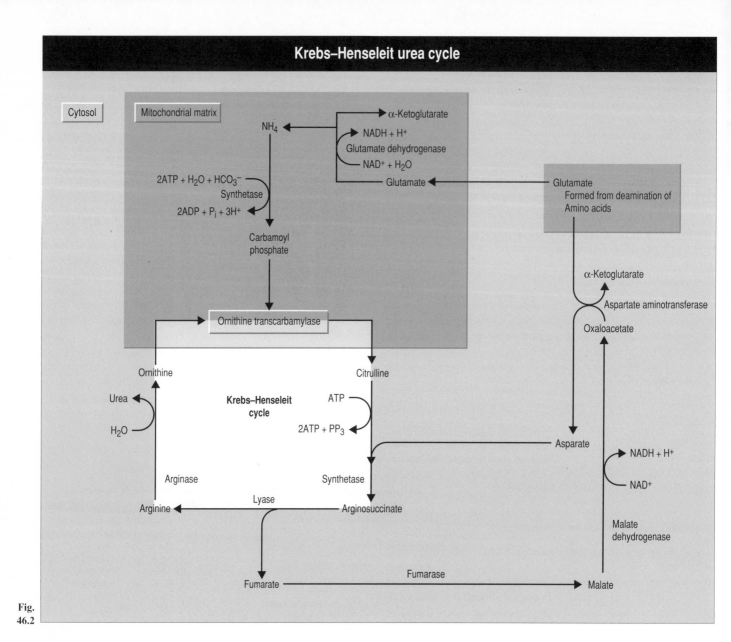

Fig.
46.2

into proteins. In phenylketonurics, the conversion of phenylalanine into tyrosine is blocked and levels of the amino acid rise drastically in the blood and the urine. If undetected and untreated in the early stages, severe complications follow which include abnormal myelination of nerves, hyperreflexia, a low brain weight and mental retardation. These complications are in evidence in untreated 1-year-old phenylketonurics who would have seemed normal and healthy at birth. Untreated phenylketonuria is also life-shortening and will usually be fatal before the patient reaches the age of 30 years.

The phenylketonuria gene has been cloned and screening programmes have ensured that most phenylketonurics are now treated. The treatment for phenylketonuria is a diet which is low in phenlyalanine, but which still contains a sufficient amount of the amino acid for normal growth. Because of the severe nature of the effects of a raised level of phenylalanine, this dietary regime is started soon after birth.

Pernicious anaemia

In pernicious anaemia, there is a deficiency of **intrinsic factor**. Intrinsic factor is responsible for the uptake of vitamin B_{12}, also called cobalamin, from the ileum. Cobalamin is a coenzyme associated with two integral enzymes of amino acid degradation, methylmalonyl CoA mutase and cystathione synthase. The mutase enzyme converts methylmalonyl CoA to succinyl CoA and the synthase enzyme converts homocysteine (a metabolite of methionine) to cystathione. The deficiency of the coenzyme results in increased levels of the enzyme substrates methylmanolyl CoA and homocysteine. Increased levels of methylmalonyl CoA cause acidosis, and increased levels of homocysteine cause homocysteinuria.

There are also a number of defects in the metabolism of methylmalonyl CoA which result in acidosis and increased levels of methylmalonate in the urine. In approximately 50% of these patients, there is a defect in the conversion of a derivative of colbalamin to colbalamin itself. These patients respond favourably to treatment with vitamin B_{12}. Other patients have a defective enzyme involved in methylmalonyl CoA metabolism, for example methylmalonyl CoA mutase, and will not therefore respond to vitamin B_{12}.

Vitamin B_{12} is also essential in the synthesis of purines and pyrimidines and a lack of cobalamin is damaging to the haematopoietic system due to the rapid turnover of red blood cells.

47 Synthesis of amino acids

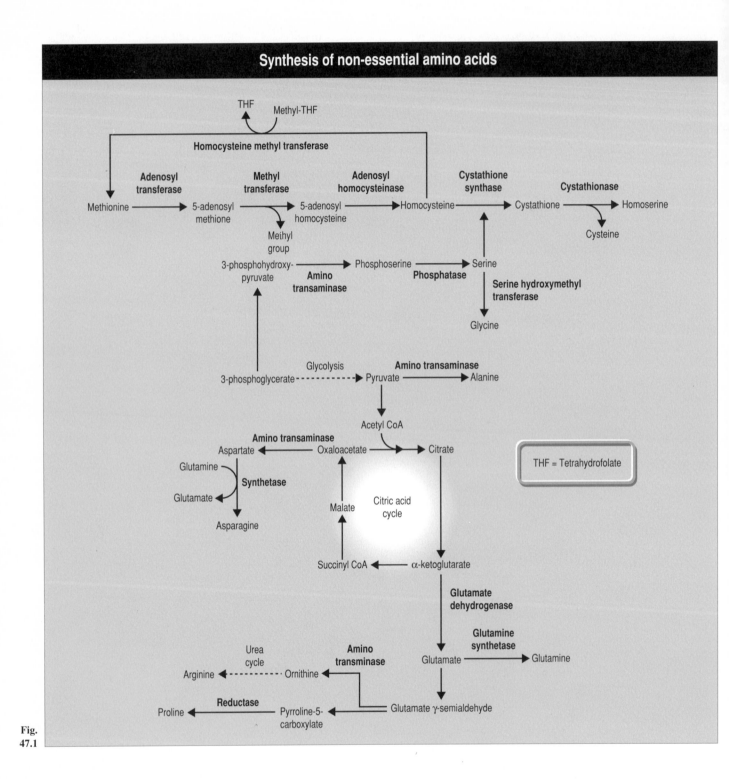

Synthesis of non-essential amino acids

Fig. 47.1

Of the 20 amino acids that exist in the body, nine cannot be synthesized and have to be obtained from the diet. These are called **essential amino acids.** The remaining 11 amino acids can be synthesized in the body and are called non-essential amino acids. This chapter will discuss the synthesis of the non-essential amino acids.

SUPPLY OF THE AMINO GROUP

In the synthesis of most amino acids, the amino group is supplied by **glutamate**. Glutamate is formed in a reaction catalysed by glutamate dehydrogenase:

$$NH_4^+ + \alpha\text{-ketoglutarate} + NADPH + H^+ \rightarrow glutamate + NADP^+ + H_2O$$

A further NH_4^+ group can be incorporated by the amination of glutamate to form glutamine. This reaction is catalysed by **glutamine synthase**:

$$NH_4^+ + glutamate + ATP \rightarrow glutamine + ADP + Pi + H^+$$

The amino group on glutamate can then be transferred to a keto-acid to form an amino acid by a transamination reaction.

Control of glutamine synthase

Glutamine synthase is a key controller in nitrogen metabolism. Glutamine is involved in the synthesis of a number of important compounds, including the amino acids **tryptophan** and **histidine**, the nucleotide **CTP** and the pyrimidine ring precursor **carbamoyl phosphate**. The final products of glutamine metabolism bind to the enzyme and inhibit its activity. The activity of glutamine synthase is also affected by the reversible covalent attachment of AMP to a tyrosine residue in the enzyme. The addition and removal of the AMP is catalysed by **adenylyl transferase** whose activity in turn is modulated by interchangeable regulator proteins. When levels of ATP or α-ketoglutarate are raised, AMP is removed from glutamine synthase, which increases its activity. When levels of glutamate or glutamine are raised, the AMP is added to the enzyme, which reduces its activity.

Synthesis of the carbon skeletons

The 11 non-essential amino acids that can be synthesized by the body are **alanine, arginine, asparagine, aspartate, cysteine, glutamine, glycine, proline, serine, glutamate and tyrosine**. The formation of all of these amino acids except for tyrosine is shown in Fig. 47.1. **Tyrosine** is formed by the hydroxylation of phenylalanine by phenylalanine hydroxylase:

$$phenylalanine + O_2 + tetrahydrobiopterin \rightarrow tyrosine + H_2O + dihydrobiopterin$$

Tetrahydrobiopterin acts as an electron carrier in this reaction and is regenerated by the reduction of dihydrobiopterin, which uses NADPH as a reductant.

Serine, **glycine** and **cysteine** are formed from an intermediate of the glycolytic pathway, 3-phosphoglycerate. The phosphatase enzyme which converts phosphoserine to serine is inhibited by serine, providing a feedback regulation for the pathway.

Glycine is formed from serine by the removal of a one-carbon unit and its attachment to a tetrahydrofolate (THF) carrier. The carbon unit is carried on either the N_5 or N_{10} nitrogen atom of THF as methylene-THF. THF can exist in a number of oxidation states depending on the carbon group carried, for example a methyl-THF donates a methyl group to homocysteine to form methionine.

An example of another carrier of carbon units is **adenosylmethionine**. This carrier has a much higher transfer potential for the release of the carbon unit than has methyl-THF, and is used to methylate a number of important molecules, e.g. noradrenaline. The formation of adenosyl-methionine forms part of a methionine salvage pathway in which methionine is regenerated by the methylation of homocysteine by methyl-THF. The enzyme that catalyses the formation of methionine from homocysteine is a methyltransferase which uses vitamin B_{12} as a coenzyme.

Cleavage of cystathione results in the formation of the amino acids **cysteine** and **homoserine**. Homoserine is then converted into ketobutyrate which is transported into the mitochondria and metabolized to succinyl CoA.

48 Integration of metabolism

Effects of insulin on adipose, liver, and muscle tissue

Increased uptake of nutrients	Glycolysis	Glycogenesis	Amino acid metabolism	Lipid metabolism
Glucose • Muscle • Adipose	Induction of hexokinase and glucokinase	Dephosphorylation and activation of glycogen synthase	Increased protein synthesis	Stimulation of lipoprotein lipase
Amino acids • Muscle	Stimulation of phosphofructokinase	Phosphorylation and activation of glycogen phosphorylation ↓ Stimulation of glycogen synthesis • Liver • Muscle	Decreased protein breakdown • Liver/muscle	Inhibition of hormone-sensitive triglyceride lipase Breakdown of blood lipids and uptake of products into adipose cells
	Inhibition of gluconeogenesis ↓ Increased rate of glycolysis • Adipose • Muscle • Liver		Excess pyruvate converted to lactate or alanine which can be transported to the liver • Muscle	Activation of pyruvate dehydrogenase and acetyl CoA carboxylase → increased fatty acid synthesis
				Inhibition of carnitine acyl transferase by malonyl CoA → reduced fatty acid breakdown
				Compensatory rise in pentose phosphate pathway • Adipose/liver

Fig. 48.1

Feeding and starvation are associated with changes in the metabolism of the body. Feeding results in a large influx of metabolic substrates into the body and the metabolism has to adapt quickly to store the nutrients as proteins, lipids and glycogen. Starvation is exactly the opposite of feeding and the metabolism of the body must be able to co-ordinate a controlled breakdown of the body's energy storage polymers to provide adequate substrates for energy generation.

FEEDING

Shortly after feeding, insulin is released into the circulation from β-cells in the islets of Langerhans of the pancreas. The overall effect of insulin on metabolism is the stimulation of biosynthetic pathways so that the digested and absorbed substrates such as glucose or amino acids can be converted into a form that can be stored. Some of the effects of insulin on metabolism have been described in earlier chapters and its overall effects are shown in Fig. 48.1.

STARVATION

There are three distinct phases through which the metabolism of the body passes when in a state of starvation: (i) the post absorptive phase; (ii) the gluconeogenic phase; and (iii) the ketotic phase. These three phases and their associated metabolic states are shown in Fig. 48.2.

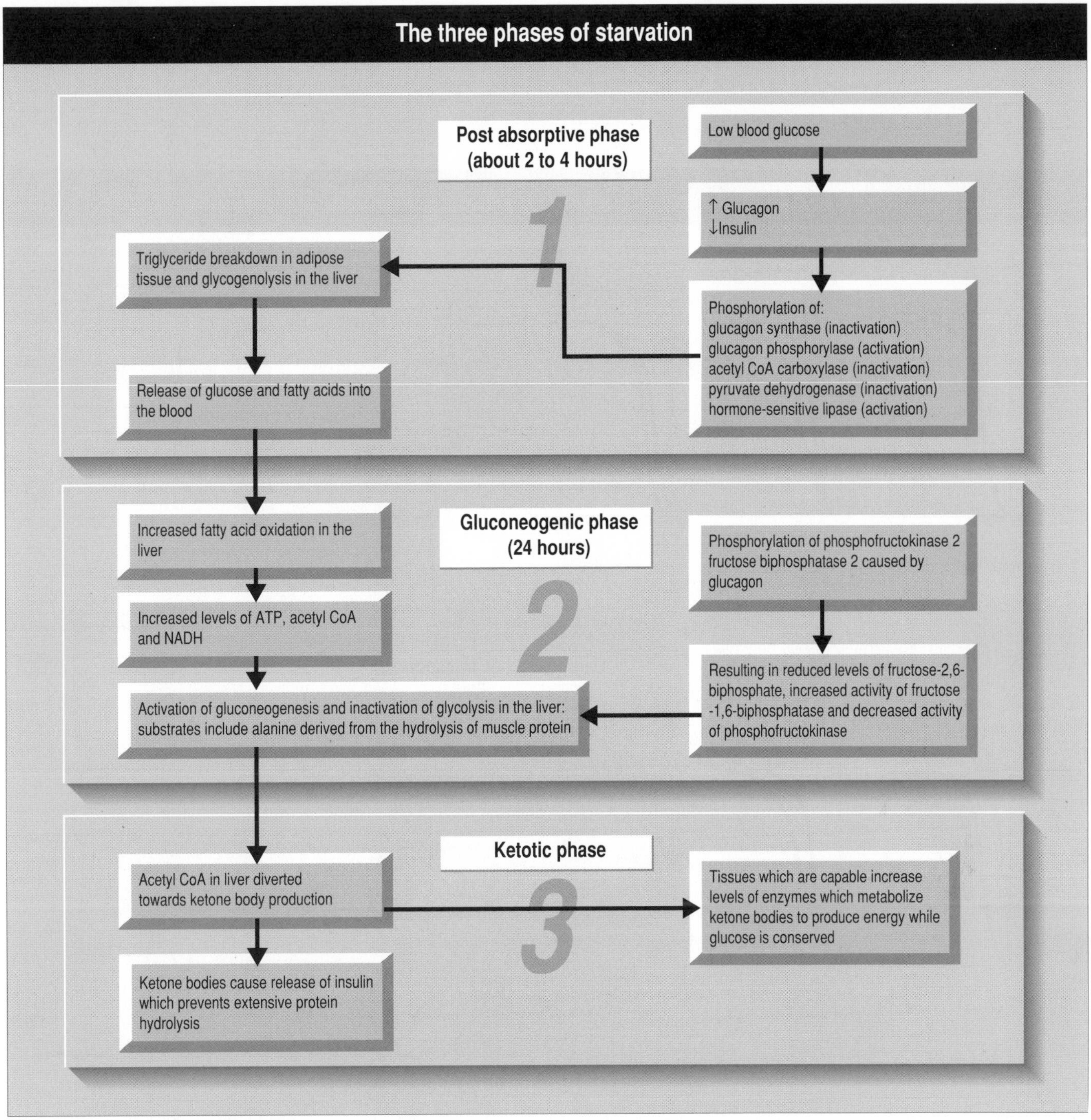

The three phases of starvation

Post absorptive phase (about 2 to 4 hours)

Low blood glucose

↑ Glucagon
↓ Insulin

Phosphorylation of:
glucagon synthase (inactivation)
glucagon phosphorylase (activation)
acetyl CoA carboxylase (inactivation)
pyruvate dehydrogenase (inactivation)
hormone-sensitive lipase (activation)

Triglyceride breakdown in adipose tissue and glycogenolysis in the liver

Release of glucose and fatty acids into the blood

1

Gluconeogenic phase (24 hours)

Increased fatty acid oxidation in the liver

Increased levels of ATP, acetyl CoA and NADH

Activation of gluconeogenesis and inactivation of glycolysis in the liver: substrates include alanine derived from the hydrolysis of muscle protein

Phosphorylation of phosphofructokinase 2 fructose biphosphatase 2 caused by glucagon

Resulting in reduced levels of fructose-2,6-biphosphate, increased activity of fructose-1,6-biphosphatase and decreased activity of phosphofructokinase

2

Ketotic phase

Acetyl CoA in liver diverted towards ketone body production

Tissues which are capable increase levels of enzymes which metabolize ketone bodies to produce energy while glucose is conserved

Ketone bodies cause release of insulin which prevents extensive protein hydrolysis

3

Fig. 48.2

The ketotic phase lasts only as long as the fatty supplies in the body can be broken down to form acetyl CoA for ketone body formation. Oxaloacetate, derived from glucose, is needed for the metabolism of ketone bodies. The glucose is, in turn, derived from the gluconeogenesis of amino acids from protein breakdown. Death eventually occurs from the extensive breakdown of functional proteins.

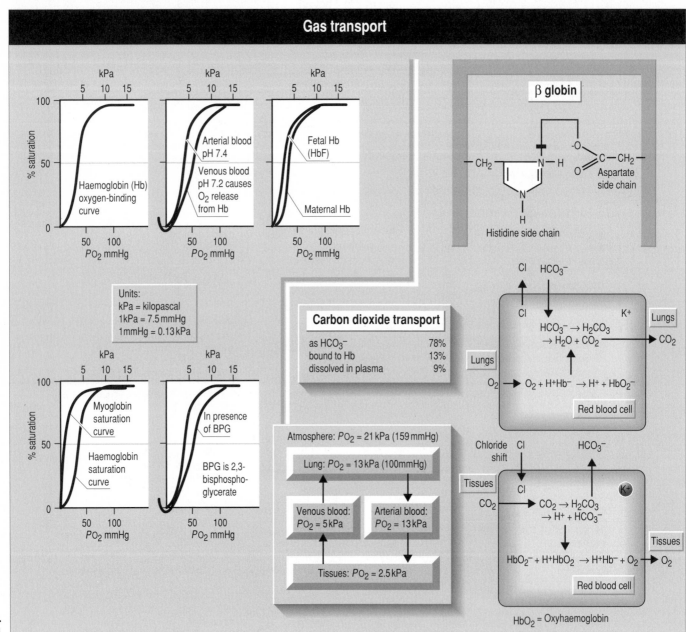

Gas transport

Fig. 49.1

TRANSPORT OF O₂ AND CO₂

In blood, most O_2 is bound to Hb. When O_2 is bound, Hb is called oxyHb. Hb is a red protein present at about 150 g/l. Each gram of Hb binds about 1.36 ml of O_2, i.e. 1 l of blood can carry about 20 ml O_2. The O_2 saturation curve for Hb is sigmoid.

Properties of the curve

The steep part of the curve lies within the range of physiological extrapulmonary PO_2 values. Therefore, a small fall in tissue PO_2 will result in a large dissociation of O_2 from Hb. The sigmoidal curve is consistent with the occurrence of co-operativity: as O_2 is taken up it increases the affinity of Hb for more O_2. At a Po_2 of 3.6 kPa, Hb is 50% saturated with O_2 (the P_{50}). A high P_{50} means a low affinity for O_2. The **Hill coefficient** for Hb is 2.8. This indicates positive co-operativity. A small shift of the curve to the right means a sharp loss of O_2 holding, and a small shift to the left implies a sharp affinity increase. Hb binds O_2 weakly at low Po_2, and tightly at high Po_2.

Hb allosterism

The binding of O_2 to Hb causes a **homotrophic** effect, when a ligand changes the affinity of another protomer of a protein for the same ligand (O_2). Hb also shows **heterotrophic** interactions, i.e. the affinity for O_2 is decreased by the binding of other ligands. Three ligands that decrease the affinity of Hb for O_2 are CO_2, H^+ ions and 2,3-bisphosphoglycerate (2,3-BPG), which occurs in red blood cells, and its net formation is a diversion from glycolysis.

CO_2 and H^+ ions

CO_2 and H^+ bind to Hb, decreasing its affinity for O_2. Conversely, when O_2 binds to Hb, it lowers Hb affinity for CO_2 and H^+ ions, and both dissociate more easily from the protein. This interaction between O_2, CO_2 and H^+ with Hb is the **Bohr effect.** In metabolically active tissues, CO_2 and H^+ concentrations are high. These bind to Hb, causing the release of O_2 to the tissues. Hb carrying CO_2 and H^+ is transported to the lung, where O_2 is taken up by free O_2-binding sites on Hb, and CO_2 and H^+ ions are released.

Transport of CO_2

CO_2 diffuses from the tissues into the blood, and into the red cells, where it is converted into carbonic acid by carbonic anhydrase:

$$CO_2 + H_2O \rightleftharpoons H_2CO_3 \rightleftharpoons HCO_3^- + H^+$$

The reaction is driven to the right because CO_2 is continuously entering the red blood cell. H^+ ions bind to Hb (releasing O_2), and HCO_3^- diffuses down a concentration gradient into the plasma in exchange for Cl^-. Thus, much CO_2 travels to the lungs as bicarbonate. Some CO_2 binds reversibly to unionized amino acid moieties on Hb promoters, forming negatively charged carbamino groups. The carbamino groups form salt bridges with groups on Hb which are positively charged, thereby promoting stability of deoxygenated Hb.

Transport of H^+ ions

H^+ ions generated in the blood must be buffered, to prevent acidosis, and H^+ binds to ionizable groups on Hb globin chains. Thus, Hb acts as a buffer. H^+ ions bind mainly to the imidazole group of C-terminal histidine residues on Hb β-chains. When O_2 dissociates from Hb, the protein polypeptide chains alter shape, bringing imidazole groups of the histidine residues close to $-COO^-$ groups of aspartate residues, and these form a non-covalent electrostatic bond which stabilizes the deoxygenated Hb. When the pH of blood falls, this shifts the O_2 saturation curve to the right, and more O_2 is released, thus increasing the buffering capacity of Hb.

In the lungs, Hb binds O_2 and changes shape. H^+ is released, and oxyHb has a negative charge. This is balanced by the positive charge of K^+ ions in the red blood cell. In other words, oxyHb acts as a stronger acid than Hb. H^+ combines with bicarbonate to form carbonic acid. Thus, the concentration of bicarbonate ions in the red blood cell is reduced, and bicarbonate ions diffuse down a concentration gradient from the plasma into the cell. To maintain electical neutrality in the cell, Cl^- ions diffuse out of the red blood cells into the plasma. This movement of Cl^- ions is termed the **chloride shift**.

In the tissues, O_2 dissociates from Hb and diffuses into the cells. Hb takes up H^+ from carbonic acid, and bicarbonate ions are formed. The negative charges of red cell bicarbonate ions are balanced by K^+ ions. Bicarbonate ions diffuse from the red cell into the plasma, and Cl^- ions diffuse from plasma into the red blood cells in exchange for bicarbonate ions. CO_2 enters the red blood cells and reacts with H_2O to form carbonic acid. Therefore, the Pco_2 within the red blood cell is kept low, and this creates a concentration gradient allowing more CO_2 to diffuse into the red blood cell from the tissues.

Effects of 2,3-BPG

2,3-BPG is present in the red blood cell in concentrations equivalent to those of Hb. 2,3-BPG binds to Hb, and shifts the O_2 saturation curve to the right. When 2,3-BPG is not bound, Hb is saturated with O_2 at the Po_2 of the tissues, and little is given up to them. 2,3-BPG is negatively charged, and binds to positive charges on the β-globin chains of the deoxygenated form of Hb, and slots into a cavity between the two chains. In the lungs, as Hb binds more O_2, the protein shape changes so that the β-globin chains move closer together and compress the sites where 2,3-BPG is bound.

FETAL Hb (HbF)

The fetus derives O_2 from the maternal circulation, and HbF has a higher affinity than does adult Hb (HbA) for O_2. HbF does not have β-chains, but γ-chains, which possess fewer positive charges in the cavity where 2,3-BPG is bound. Therefore, HbF binds 2,3-BPG less tightly than does HbA.

50 Haemoglobin

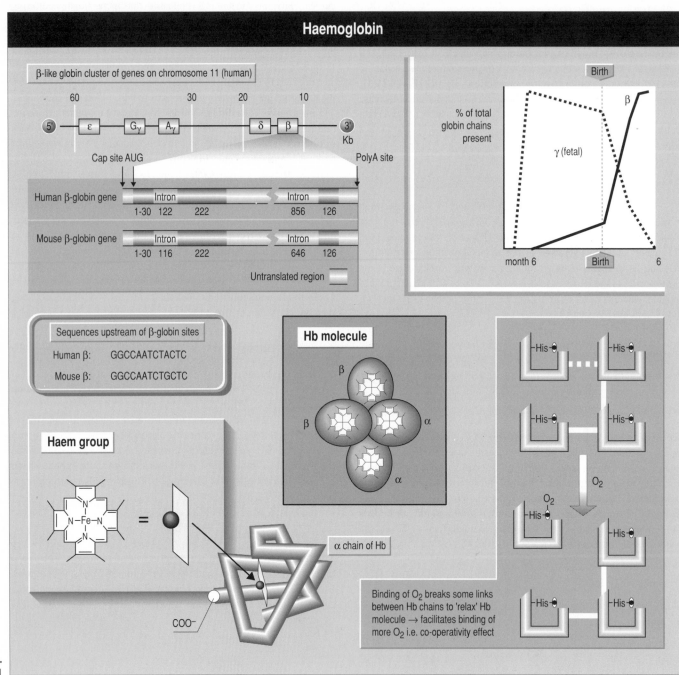

Fig. 50.1

β-GLOBIN FAMILY

Several different forms of β-like globins are formed during embryogenesis and adult life in humans and other vertebrates. In humans, these include β-, δ-, A_γ-, G_γ- and ε-globins. The genes coding for the polypeptide chains occur relatively close together on chromosome 11, and express chains which are very similar in sequence identity. Only the β- and δ-chains continue to be expressed after 6 months of postnatal life in humans.

STRUCTURE OF Hb

Hb consists of **four subunits.** Each is a globin molecule containing a **haem group,** and the four subunits are held together by non-covalent bonds. **HbA** consists of two α-chains, each 141 amino acids long, and two β-chains, each 146 amino acids long. There is a high degree of uniformity in tertiary structure among the different subunits of Hb, and each chain is arranged in multiple α-helix regions interrupted by turns of the polypeptide chain that force the subunit into a spherical shape.

THE HAEM GROUP

Each subunit of Hb contains a prosthetic haem group. Haem consists of a polyringed **porphyrin** molecule, with an atom of iron (Fe) in the ferrous (Fe(II)) form at its centre. Hb and myoglobin porphyrin is termed protoporphyrin IX. The Fe is bound to the four N atoms of the haem, but is situated outside the plane of the molecule because it is larger than the space between the N atoms. The Fe is also bound to the peptide chain of the subunit through a linkage with one of the histidine (His) residues.

Combination of Hb with O_2

O_2 can combine reversibly with each of the four subunits of Hb. The O_2 binds to the Fe atom on the face of the haem group opposite to that bound to the protein. The first O_2 binds to Fe in an α-subunit. This overcomes a repulsion between a His residue and the porphyrin ring, and allows Fe to move into the plane of the ring. At the same time, several of the ionic bonds linking amino acid residues rupture. This causes a conformational change over the whole Hb molecule. The two ß-subunits move closer to each other, although they do not actually touch. This forces the dissociation of 2,3-BPG. As the β-subunits move closer together, the two α-chains move further apart, and this makes it easier for O_2 molecules to gain access to the haem sites. Thus, as succeeding O_2 molecules bind, so they open or 'relax' the Hb molecule further, and this increases the apparent affinity of the molecule for O_2; the fourth O_2 molecule finds it easiest to bind, i.e. has the highest apparent affinity for Hb.

MYOGLOBIN

Myoglobin is a protein in muscle cells. Like Hb, it binds O_2 but, unlike Hb, myoglobin consists of a single polypeptide chain, 153 amino acids long, with one haem group which binds only one molecule of O_2. Its saturation curve is therefore not sigmoidal.

Functionally, myoglobin provides a binding site for O_2 that can be utilized by the metabolically very active skeletal and cardiac muscle fibres. Together, these two tissues account for about 30% of the O_2 consumption of the human body at rest. The saturation curve for myoglobin, over most of its length, lies to the left of that for Hb. In other words, it has a higher affinity for O_2 than has Hb. Therefore, in the tissues such as muscle, where the P_{O_2} is about 2.5–3.5 kPa, when Hb is less than 50% saturated with O_2, myoglobin is fully saturated. When the tissues demand more O_2, the P_{O_2} drops to less than 0.2 kPa, and at this order of magnitude, myoglobin releases most of its bound O_2. Unlike Hb, the binding of O_2 by myoglobin is not influenced by 2,3-BPG concentrations, CO_2 or H^+.

PATHOPHYSIOLOGY OF Hb

Hb is associated with several disease states.

Quantitative determinants

Patients may present with a red blood cell (RBC) count in the normal range, but with a mean cell volume (MCV) outside the normal range (**microcytosis**), abnormal mean cell Hb content (MCH) and abnormal mean cell Hb concentration (MCHC; **hypochromia**). This is **microcytic anaemia**, although in other forms of anaemia the patient may present with a lowered RBC count.

The anaemia may be caused by a dietary shortage of the Fe required for haem synthesis. Individuals at risk include women who are pregnant, menstruating or lactating, and vegetarians, especially vegans.

Microcytic anaemia may result from a failure to utilize Fe. Individuals at risk include those exposed to toxic substances such as lead, which block –SH groups of enzymes that catalyse reactions involved in the synthesis of haem.

Chemicals can cause a quantitative reduction in available Hb. For example, inhalation of carbon monoxide (CO), can be fatal. The CO forms a stable, bright red complex with the haem group and does not dissociate. Another example is the oxidation of the Fe(II) to Fe(III), to form **methaemoglobin**. Methaemoglobin may be formed through hereditary defects in globin synthesis, or through oxidizing compounds. In the Fe(III) states, O_2 is not bound, and, when present together with normal HbA, methaemoglobin shifts the O_2 saturation curve of the HbA to the left, making its bound O_2 less accessible to the tissues.

Qualitative determinants

In **sickle cell anaemia** patients synthesize **HbS**, an aberrant form of HbA, in which a non-polar valine (Val) residue replaces a polar glutamate residue at position six on the β-subunit ($Glu_{6\beta}$). $Glu_{6\beta}$ lies on the outer surface of HbA, and in the deoxy state of Hb, the non-polar Val residue forms hydrophobic bonds with other HbS molecules, which causes polymerization and precipitation of Hb inside the RBC. Consequently, the RBC assumes a characteristic sickle shape, and loses elasticity, which results in blockage of the microcirculation by the cells.

51 Molecular chaperones

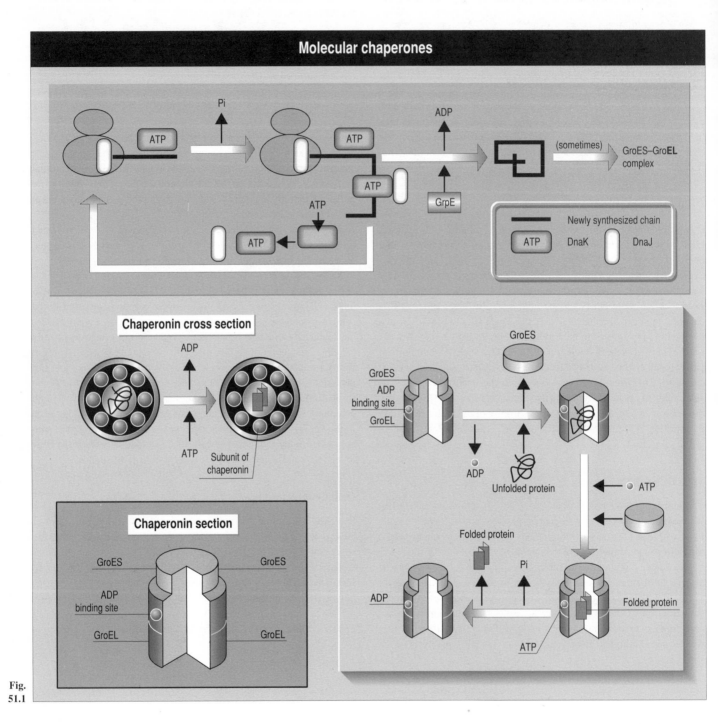

Molecular chaperones

Newly synthesized chain
ATP   DnaK   DnaJ

GroES–GroEL complex

Chaperonin cross section

Subunit of chaperonin

Chaperonin section

GroES   GroES
ADP binding site
GroEL   GroEL

GroES
ADP binding site
GroEL

Unfolded protein

Folded protein

Folded protein

Fig. 51.1

Molecular chaperones regulate the **folding** of many newly synthesized proteins. The chaperones bind newly synthesized proteins, preventing them from aggregating in the cell, and mediate protein folding into their native state. There are several, structurally unrelated families of molecular chaperones. The term 'molecular chaperone' was originally applied to the proteins nucleoplasmin and the chloroplast ribulose biphosphate carboxylase, which promote the assembly of nucleosomes. The molecular chaperones can organize themselves into structures, called **chaperonins**, which contain a central cavity in which an unfolded protein is shielded from the cell.

PRINCIPLES OF CHAPERONE ACTION

Molecular chaperones bind and stabilize proteins in their non-native form, and release them in such a way as to facilitate their folding. They can recognize structural features of proteins in their unfolded form, in particular certain amino acid sequences, but cannot bind folded proteins.

Newly formed proteins extend from the polysomes, amino-terminus leading, as unfolded peptide chains. These cannot start folding until a critical length has been reached: about 100 amino acids. These form a **protein domain**, which facilitates the further folding of the entire protein in a co-operative manner. When the chain is elongated, its hydrophobic residues are repelled by the aqueous environment and tend to bury themselves within the protein. Since so many different proteins are being synthesized simultaneously, hydrophobic residues from different chains could interact to form aggregates, and this has been shown to happen *in vitro* in the absence of molecular chaperones.

Molecular chaperones protect the nascent protein from these interactions by shielding hydrophobic surfaces during peptide elongation, and possibly also during the folding process and during translocation of the protein across membranes, and by binding the completely synthesized, but as yet unfolded protein, and allowing it to fold unhindered by the other cellular processes going on around it.

HSP

HSP60 and HSP70

The principle of molecular chaperones may provide a clue as to why HSP are produced during cellular injury or disease. It is known that the HSP70 proteins can bind proteins **after** they have been incompletely denatured during cellular distress. Therefore, they may provide a means of protecting the cell from undergoing massive protein aggregation.

HSP70 proteins comprise two functional domains: (i) a polypeptide-binding domain at the carboxy terminal; and (ii) a nucleotide-binding site at the amino terminal. There is evidence that ATP is bound and hydrolysed to ADP at the amino terminal of HSP70, and this provides the energy to induce a conformational change in HSP70 that results in the release of the folded polypeptide.

Action of HSP70

The mechanism whereby HSP70 proteins act in concert to regulate protein folding and release in *Escherichia coli* cytosol has been partially elucidated. There are at least five proteins in the cytosol that mediate protein folding, namely **DnaK**, **DnaJ**, **GrpE**, **GroEL** and **GroES**. They regulate the folding of newly synthesized proteins, and may also protect already folded proteins during periods of cellular stress. They have already been shown to inhibit the heat denaturation of a heat-labile protein, luciferase, produced by fireflies. The steps in protein folding are the following.

1 DnaJ and Dnak, with bound ATP attached to it, bind the unfolded polypeptide chain as it is formed by the ribosome, and the bound ATP is hydrolysed to ADP.

2 DnaJ and DnaK bind to each other as the polypeptide starts to fold, and the DnaK–ADP–DnaJ–polypeptide complex is stabilized.

3 The protein GrpE promotes the dissociation of ADP from DnaK, perhaps by binding to the site where ADP is bound. ATP binds to its site on DnaK, and the folded polypeptide is released.

4 In some cases, the released protein is bound by GroEL, which, through an ATP-dependent interaction with GroES, permits protein folding to be completed.

CHAPERONINS

The term 'chaperonins' has been given to the **HSP60** protein family. The term describes a quaternary structure of proteins which assemble to form a compartment in which newly synthesized proteins can fold, protected from other folding proteins, thus eliminating the risk of protein aggregation. Analysis of chaperonins has revealed structures consisting of 14 subunits, stacked in two heptameric rings with a central cavity, which can hold proteins of up to about 90 kDa in size. In *E. coli*, the chaperonins are made up of two HSP60 proteins, GroEL and GroES. The newly synthesized proteins are held in the chaperonin in what has been called a 'molten globule' state. The term describes partially folded proteins whose hydrophobic surfaces have not yet become totally buried in the protein. GroEL and GroES interact via a sequence of ATP binding and hydrolysis, which provide the energy for the binding and release of the folded protein.

Eukaryotic chaperones and chaperonins

In yeast cells, molecular chaperones have been described whose function is to assist in the transfer of proteins across the mitochondrial membrane. Proteins formed in the cytosol must first be unfolded before they can cross the mitochondrial membrane, and refolded once they have done so. This is accomplished through the action of mitochondrial molecular chaperones. There is evidence that proteins in the cytosol are held in an unfolded state by HSP70 proteins, and the energy for this is provided by ATP. The polypeptide chain passes through the lipid bilayer of the mitochondrial membrane, and on the inner surface the polypeptide chain is folded under the direction of HSP70, acting together with HSP60.

A number of other chaperonins have now been described, including one found in eukaryotic cytosols, called **TCP-1**, or **CCT** (also called chaperonin of eukaryotic cytosol), which is particularly abundant in developing embryos, testis and lymphoid tissue. It has been shown that disruption of yeast chaperonins are lethal for the cell.

Abbreviations

A	adenine		GTP	guanosine triphosphate
ACP	acyl carrier protein		GTPase	guanosine triphosphatase
ACTH	adrenocorticotrophin		H_2	hydrogen
ADP	adenosine diphosphate		H_2CO_3	hydrogen carbonate
AMP	adenosine monophosphate		H_2O	water
ATP	adenosine triphosphate		H_2O_2	hydrogen peroxide
ATPase	adenosine triphosphatase		H_3PO_4	phosphoric acid
bp	base pairs		Hb	haemoglobin
2,3-BPG	2,3-bisphosphoglycerate		HbA	adult Hb
C	cytosine		HbF	fetal Hb
Ca	calcium		HDL	high-density lipoprotein
$CaCl_2$	calcium chloride		hfr	high frequency of recombination
cAMP	cyclic AMP		Hg	mercury
CAP	catabolic activator protein		HGPRTase	hypoxanthine–guanine phosphoribosyl transferase
CCK	cholecystokinin		HIV	human immunodeficiency virus
cDNA	complementary DNA		hnRNA	heterogeneous nuclear RNA
CDP	cytidine triphosphate		HRE	hormone response elements
cGMP	cyclic guanosine monophosphate		HSP	heat shock protein
CGRP	calcitonin gene-related peptide		Hyp	hydroxyproline
CH_3COOH	acetic acid		I	inosinic acid
CH_3COONa	sodium acetate		ICF	intracellular fluid
Cl_2	chlorine		IDL	intermediate density lipoprotein
CO	carbon monoxide		IF	initiation factor
CO_2	carbon dioxide		IgA	immunoglobulin A
CoA	coenzyme A		IGF	insulin-like growth factor
–COOH	carboxyl group		Il-1	interleukin 1
CRS	cytokine receptor superfamily		IMP	inosine monophosphate
CTP	cytidine triphosphate		IP_3	inositol trisphosphate
cyt	cytochrome		IRS-1	insulin receptor substrate 1
d	2′-deoxyribo-		JAK	Janus kinase
Da	dalton		K	potassium
DAG	diacylglycerol		K_m	Michaelis constant
dCTP	deoxycytidine triphosphate		LDL	low-density lipoprotein
dd	dideoxynucleotide		LTR	long terminal repeats
DFP	di-isopropylphosphofluoridate		MAPK	mitogen-activated protein kinase
DHT	5α-dihydrotestosterone		MCH	mean cell Hb content
DNA	deoxyribonucleic acid		MCV	mean cell volume
DNAase	deoxyribonuclease		Mg	magnesium
dTTP	deoxythymidine triphosphate		MGE	mobile genetic element
dUDP	deoxyuridine diphosphate		MCHC	mean corpuscular Hb concentration
dUTPase	deoxyuridine triphosphatase		MMTV	mouse mammary tumour virus
ECF	extracellular fluid		Mn	manganese
EF	elongation factor		mRNA	messenger RNA
EGF	epidermal growth factor		Na	sodium
emf	electromotive force		NADH	nicotinamide adenine dinucleotide
ER	endoplasmic reticulum		$NADP^+$	nicotinamide adenine dinucleotide phosphate
FAD	flavine adenine dinucleotide		–NH_2	amino group
Fe	iron		O_2	oxygen
FGF	fibroblast growth factor		–OH	hydroxyl group
fMET	formyl methionine		^{32}P	phosphorus-32
GDP	guanosine diphosphate		Pa	pascal
GH	growth hormone		PCR	polymerase chain reaction
GMP	guanosine monophosphate		PDGF	platelet-derived growth factor

PFK	phosphofructokinase		UMP	uridine monophosphate
Pi	inorganic phosphate		UTP	uridine triphosphate
PIP$_2$	phosphatidylinositol-4,5-biphosphate		UV	ultraviolet
PKC	protein kinase C		VLDL	very low-density lipoprotein
PLA$_2$	phospholipase A$_2$		Zn	zinc
PLC	phospholipase C			
PLP	pyridoxal phosphate			
PRPP	5-phosphoribosyl-1-pyrophosphate		**Amino acid abbreviations**	
R	gas constant		Ala	alanine
RBC	red blood cell		Arg	arginine
RF	release factor		Asn	asparagine
RNA	ribonucleic acid		Asp	aspartate
RNAase	ribonuclease		Cys	cysteine
rRNA	ribosomal RNA		Gln	glutamine
RTF	resistance transfer factor		Glu	glutamate
S	Svedberg unit		Gly	glycine
scRNA	small cytoplasmic RNA		His	histidine
snRNA	small nuclear RNA		Ile	isoleucine
SRP	signal recognition particle		Leu	leucine
STATS	signal transducers and transcription activators		Lys	lysine
T	thymine		Met	methionine
TGF	transforming growth factor		Phe	phenylalanine
THF	tetrahydrofolate		Pro	proline
TMP	thymidine monophosphate		Ser	serine
tRNA	transfer RNA		Thr	threonine
TPP	thymine pyrophosphate		Trp	tryptophan
U	uracil		Tyr	tyrosine
UDP	uridine diphosphate		Val	valine

Glossary

A site ribosomal recognition site where next mRNA codon is exposed to incoming tRNA

activation energy critical energy level for chemical reaction to occur

active transport energy-requiring movement of substances across biomembranes

affinity strength of attraction between two binding sites

agonist ligand that triggers a response (see **ligand**)

allele alternative form of a gene that can occupy a chromosomal genetic locus

allosteric proteins can alter binding site properties in response to ligand occupancy at another site

amphipathic molecule possessing both hydrophilic and hydrophobic properties

anaemic deficient in haemoglobin

anion negatively charged ion

annealing two complementary nucleic acid strands joining

antibody immunoglobulin produced in response to an antigen, which binds it

anticodon set of three consecutive tRNA bases complementary to a mRNA codon

antigen substance, usually foreign to body, that provokes antibody formation

antimetabolite substance blocking a metabolic (usually enzyme) reaction

antiporter membrane protein transporting substance across membrane with simultaneous transport of another substance the opposite way

autocrine hormonal action on cell by substance produced by the same cell

autosomal recessive Mendelian recessive genetic inheritance carried on an autosome

autosome chromosome other than sex chromosome

avian referring to birds

bacteriophage virus that infects bacteria

base proton (H^+) acceptor in solution, e.g. purines, pyrimidines

benign medically, a non-cancerous tumour that does not invade other tissues or destroy any healthy tissue

C terminal free $-COO^-$ group at end of a polypeptide chain

cap-binding protein binds to cap region of mRNA; required for initiation of eukaryotic transcription

carcinogen agent that may cause cancer

cardiotonic heart stimulant

cation positively charged ion

cDNA library collection of DNA strands complementary to source tissue DNA

chi sequence repeated short DNA sequence on bacterial chromosome where RecA-mediated recombination is stimulated

chondroblast cartilage cell producing cartilage matrix

cloning producing identical cells or molecules from single starting cell or molecule

co-operative binding ligand binds to protein and changes affinity for other sites for the same ligand on the protein

codon set of three consecutive bases on DNA or RNA, specifying an amino acid or a signal for the end of translation

coenzyme (cofactor) non-protein required by a protein for bioactivity

cofactor see **coenzyme**

conformation three-dimensional arrangement

constitutive gene a gene continuously expressed without the need for a transcription initiation factor

control element a DNA sequence that influences the expression of nearby genes

cosmid a cloning vector plasmid containing phage λ *cos* sequences

cotransport linked transport of substances across a biomembrane

crista mitochondrial inner membrane infolding

crossover exchange of genes between homologous chromosomes during meiosis

cytoskeleton internal protein skeleton of eukaryotic cell

cytosol soluble cytoplasmic compartment

degenerate one amino acid can be encoded by several different codons

dimer protein formed of two subunits

diploid organism whose cell has two sets of chromosomes

docking protein protein that 'places' another in its binding site

domain structurally defined membrane or chromatin region, or globular region of a protein

electrochemical gradient transmembrane gradient defined by ionic and electrical gradients

endocrine ductless glandular function

enhancer a DNA control site in eukaryotic genes, whose activation by specific proteins increases transcription of the gene

eukaryote organism whose cells have bounded nuclei containing organized chromatin and cytoskeletons

exocytosis secretion of chemicals from eukaryotic cells

exon DNA sequence unit coding for part of a polypeptide, or for rRNA or tRNA

facilitated diffusion membrane transport down a concentration gradient utilizing a carrier system, but no energy

familial traits found in some families; not necessarily inherited

fibril thread-like component of a fibre

fibroblast connective tissue cell

flip-flop transition of a lipid or protein from one membrane surface to the other

G protein guanine nucleotide-binding protein on cytoplasmic surface of cell membrane, forming part of hormone signalling to target cell

genetic recombination meiotic exchange of DNA between homologous chromosomes during gamete formation in sexually reproducing organisms

genome genetic database of a single organism or cell

genomic library collection of DNA chromosomal fragments from one genome

globin protein constituent of haemoglobin

glucocorticoids adrenal steroids influencing carbohydrate metabolism; some are anti-inflammatory

glycosides compounds which when hydrolysed yield a sugar and a non-sugar, e.g. digoxin

glycosylation formation of eukaryotic glycoproteins through addition of oligosaccharide side chain to protein

growing fork locus in DNA replication

haploid cell or organism having one set of chromosomes

helical spiral chain arrangement of protein or nucleic acid molecules forming rod-like helix

hepatocyte liver cell

heterogeneous having dissimilar components

heterotrophic effects allosteric effects due to interactions between different ligands

homodimer protein consisting of two identical subunits

homologous resembling in origin and structure

homotrophic effects allosteric effects due to interactions between identical ligands

hormone response element (HRE) region of DNA that binds hormone–receptor complex

hydrolysis addition of OH^- and H^+ ions of H_2O to a molecule which is consequently split into simpler molecules

hydrophilic water attracting

hydrophobic water repelling

in vitro in test tubes ('in glass')

inducer chemical or physical stimulus to gene expression or enzyme action

intercalate to slip between adjacent bases in DNA

intron non-coding region of DNA that may be transcribed but later spliced out of mRNA

isoelectric pH pH at which protein is uncharged

isomer compound chemically identical to others, but with different spatial arrangement, e.g. stereoisomer

Klenow fragment fragment of DNA polymerase I, containing all the $3' \rightarrow 5'$ exonuclease and polymerase activity

lap-joint intermediate hybrid in genetic recombination

ligand a molecule that binds to another with functional purpose

lipids class of hydrophobic compounds including fats, phospholipids and steroids

lipoprotein compound composed of protein and lipid

lumen internal space of subcellular organelle or of sac-like or tubular organ

malignant tumour that destroys tissue of origin or invades and destroys other tissues

matrix medium or ground substance of tissues

meiosis nuclear division producing haploid daughter cells from diploid parent cell

metastasis spread of cancerous cells to other tissues

micelle spherical ordered arrangement of molecules such as phospholipids in aqueous medium

mitosis nuclear division, when daughter cells have identical chromosomal complement as parent

mobile genetic element DNA sequence able to be inserted on same or other chromosomes and alter gene expression (also called transposable element)

monomer molecule composed of a single unit

mutagenic able to cause a mutation

mutation change in nature or composition of DNA resulting in change in characteristics of gene expression in cell

N terminal amino terminus of polypeptide chain

nascent newly synthesized; not yet active

nonsense codon a termination codon

Okazaki fragments short DNA sequences formed on lagging ($3' \rightarrow 5'$) strand during discontinuous DNA replication

oligomer molecule composed of a few monomer units

oncogene gene carried by cancer cell or virus, that is partly or wholly responsible for tumour formation

operon prokaryotic genetic unit in which several genes are clustered and transcribed into polycistronic mRNA

organelle functional structure within a eukaryotic cell

osteoblast bone-forming cell

P site ribosomal site where the last mRNA codon was read (see also **A site**)

palindrome sequence reading the same both ways, e.g. in DNA: AACAA

paracrine local hormone acting on neighbouring cells

passive transport simple diffusion down a concentration gradient; includes facilitated diffusion

pentose a monosaccharide with formula $(CH_2O)_5$, e.g. ribose

phage see **bacteriophage**

phasmid vector consisting of a combination of a plasmid with phage λ

phenotype biochemical and physical characteristics of an organism

pinocytosis uptake of liquid into the cell

plasmid circular bacterial or yeast DNA replicating independently of chromosomes

polycistronic mRNA codes for more than one polypeptide

polymer macromolecule consisting of several similar or identical subunits

polysaccharide macromolecular carbohydrate polymers, e.g. glycogen

polysome ribosomal aggregate on mRNA during translation

primer short fragment of RNA necessary to initiate DNA polymerase action

primosome prepriming protein assembly necessary for primer synthesis

prohormone hormone precursor

prokaryote unicellular organisms, e.g. bacteria, lacking membrane-bounded nucleus and other organelles such as mitochondria

promoter DNA sequence necessary for initiation of transcription

proofreading property of DNA polymerase to detect base mismatches

prosthetic group non-protein moiety, e.g. haem, forming part of protein active site

protomer inactive enzyme form

proton H^+ (H_3O^+ in some texts)

purine base, commonly adenine or guanine in nucleic acids

pyrimidine base, commonly cytosine, thymine or uracil in nucleic acids

receptor protein that recognizes a ligand, and that constitutes the primary member in the chain of communication between ligand and cell

receptor antagonist ligand that binds receptor, blocks agonist binding and produces no response

receptor superfamily group of intracellular receptors, with structural similarities, which act as transcription activators, e.g. glucocorticoid and retinoic acid receptors

recombination exchange of DNA between homologous chromosomes during meiosis

replication fork Y-shaped point where DNA is unwound and simultaneously replicated

replicon unit of DNA that replicates sequentially and contains an origin of replication

replisome protein assembly on DNA, needed for replication

repressor bacterial protein that binds to the operon to repress transcription

resistance transfer factor (RTF) factor on plasmid that enables transfer of drug resistance to another bacterial cell

second messenger intracellular chemical signal synthesized in response to stimulation of receptor on cell membrane

sedimentation coefficient estimate of size of macromolecule from its rate of sedimentation in a sucrose gradient

semi-conservative replication means of DNA replication

sex pilus means of transmitting F factors from one bacterium to another

Shine–Dalgarno sequence bacterial mRNA 5′-AGGAGG-3′ sequence before initiation codon

signal sequence temporary hydrophobic sequence of amino acids at amino terminal, important for transfer of secretory products across membranes

SOS response sequence of repair responses in *E. coli* in response to damage stimuli

splicing cutting nucleic acid in order to insert sequences, thus creating recombinant nucleic acid

splicosome assembly of ribonucleoprotein that splices RNA

stop signal signal that stops macromolecular elongation

supercoiling twisting of the double helix on itself

symport simultaneous, linked transport of two molecules across a biomembrane, both in the same direction

template pattern from which a molecule is synthesized, e.g. DNA strand is a template for its replication

transcription synthesis of complementary RNA from DNA .

transition DNA base substitution causing mutation

translation protein synthesis by ribosomes on mRNA template

translocation removal of part of a chromosome to another, non-homologous chromosome

transposable element see **mobile genetic element**

transposition replication of a DNA sequence on one chromosome in another chromosome

transposon replicated transposed sequence

transversion substitution of a pyrimidine for a purine or vice versa

Uniport membrane transport of a molecule by a membrane protein

van der Waals forces weak form of non-covalent bonding between neutral molecules

vector agent that carries a message, e.g. plasmid, bacteriophage

zwitterion ion with negative and positive charges, e.g. amino acids

Sources

Baulieu, E–E. & Kelly, P.A. (Eds) (1990) *Hormones From Molecules to Disease*. Hermann Publishers in Arts and Science, Chapman and Hall, New York, USA.

Darnell, J., Lodish, H. & Baltimore, D. (1986) *Molecular Cell Biology*. Scientific American Books, New York, USA.

Devlin, T.M. (Ed.) (1992) *Textbook of Biochemistry*, 3rd edn. Wiley-Liss, New York, USA.

Greenstein, B.D. (1994) *Endocrinology at a Glance*. Blackwell Scientific Publications, Oxford, UK.

Lawrence, E. (Ed.)(1989) *Hendersons Dictionary of Biological Terms*, 10th edn. Longmans Scientific and Technical, Essex, England.

Liptrot, G.F., Thompson, J.J. & Walker, G.R. (1986) *Modern Physical Chemistry*, 4th edn. Bell and Hyman Ltd., London.

Martin, E.A. (Ed.) (1987) *Oxford Reference Concise Medical Dictionary*, 2nd edn. Oxford University Press, Oxford, UK.

Old, R.W. & Primrose, S.B. (1994) *Principles of Gene Manipulation*, 5th edn. Blackwell Scientific Publications, Oxford, UK.

Parker, M.G. (Ed.) (1993) *Steroid Hormone Action*. IRL Press at Oxford University Press, Oxford, UK.

Robbins, R.S., Kumar, V. & Robbins S.L. (1989) *Robbins Pathologic Basis of Disease*, 4th Edn. W.B. Saunders Company Philadelphia, USA.

Salway, J.G. (1994) *Metabolism at a Glance*, Blackwell Scientific Publications, Oxford, UK.

Sambrook, J., Fritsch, E.F. & Maniatis, (1989). *Molecular Cloning. A Laboratory Manual*. 2nd edn. Cold Spring Harbor Laboratory Press, USA.

Segel, I.H. (1968) *Biochemical Calculations*, John Wiley & Sons Inc., USA.

Stryer, L. (1988) *Biochemistry*, 3rd edn. W.H. Freeman and Company, New York, USA.

Trends in Biochemical Sciences (1994) **19(1)**, Inactivation of MAP kinases, pp. 1–2; Hsp chaperones, pp. 20–25.

Trends in Biochemical Sciences (1994) **19(2)**, Model of protein kinase C isotype, pp. 73–77; Mitochondrial yeast chaperones pp. 87–92.

Trends in Biochemical Sciences (1994) **19(5)**, Cytokine receptor superfamily pp. 222–227.

Trends in Biochemical Sciences (1994) **19(7)**, IRS–1 signalling system pp. 289–293.

Trends in Biochemical Sciences (1994) **19(12)**, Chaperonins pp. 543–548.

Weatherall, D.J. (1991) *The New Genetics and Clinical Practice*. 3rd edn. Oxford University Press, Oxford, UK.

Index